# EDUCATING HEARING-IMPAIRED CHILDREN IN ORDINARY SCHOOLS

# Educating
# Hearing-impaired Children
# in Ordinary Schools

*by*
## J. C. JOHNSON
B.A., Dip.Ed.Psych.

*Department of Audiology and Education of the Deaf*
*University of Manchester*

*With a Foreword by*
## SIR ALEXANDER EWING

MANCHESTER UNIVERSITY PRESS

Printed in Great Britain by Butler & Tanner Ltd., Frome and London

# FOREWORD

THE specific research that Mr. Johnson has reported in this book grew out of a major collaborative project which was begun a number of years ago and is still in progress. The chief aim of the project is to find all children in the administrative county of Cheshire who are in any way handicapped by hearing impairment and to study their mental growth and social development in relation to their deafness. Such a survey has been made possible by the very full co-operation of the County Medical Officer of Health and his staff with ourselves in the Department of Audiology and Education of the Deaf in the University of Manchester.

A special feature of the project is the holding of joint clinical sessions to provide audiological testing with medical examinations and consequent case conferences about each child who is seen. At four of the county audiology clinics either Mr. J. M. Kodicek, F.R.C.S., or Dr. O. T. Taylor are always present at joint sessions to make ear, nose and throat examinations, diagnose deafness and recommend medical or surgical treatment where they find it to be advisable. One or both of the county's peripatetic teachers of the deaf attend all sessions and report on hearing-impaired pupils in ordinary schools to whom they give part-time educational treatment and to receive medical and audiological information that is relevant to their responsibilities. This is an extension, in principle, of a long-established practice of holding joint clinical sessions in the University with the co-operation of Professor V. F. Lambert, Director of the Department of Otolaryngology, and his staff, in particular Mr. K. Harrison, F.R.C.S.

From our Cheshire Survey and from other sources we have learnt that the problems of educating hearing-impaired pupils in ordinary schools involve a considerable number of children. At the time of writing this foreword, 242 Cheshire children are included in the survey, in addition to 99 of pre-school age and 109 who are pupils in special schools for the deaf or partially deaf.

v

Month by month it is found that there are more partially deaf children who should be added to the case lists.

Mr. J. C. Johnson's most valuable contribution has been that of an experienced educational psychologist who undertook an intensive study of 68 cases and a review of the whole background to the subject. He has made it clear that the problem is a national one involving many of our children. In this book he has reported great variations in the educational attainment of hearing-impaired children that are not at all closely correlated with the degree and nature of their deafness. He has made it clear that in cases in which communication difficulties result in undue mental stress, emotional and social development is at stake. His emphasis on the great importance of the detection, diagnosis and treatment of deafness in the pre-school stage continues to be supported by the findings of other researchers as they complete their investigations. That is true also of his recommendations for the training and appointment by local authorities of more qualified audiologists.

By making this book so concise and readable, Mr. Johnson has presented his data in a form accessible to administrators, as well as to audiologists, educationalists, psychologists, otolaryngologists, paediatricians and others whose team-work is necessary to efficient management of deafness in childhood. The book is published at a time when national provision for partially deaf children is being extended. It is made clear that the advantages and disadvantages of alternative forms of provision and their suitability in individual cases need to be kept under constant and thorough review.

Very grateful acknowledgments are due to the Trustees of the Nuffield Foundation for having made this research possible and to Mr. Johnson for carrying it out. We are particularly indebted to Dr. Arnold Brown and his staff, including Dr. N. Robertshaw, for the excellent efficiency of their co-operation.

A. W. G. EWING

Department of Audiology and Education of the Deaf,
    University of Manchester.
    *2nd November 1961*

# ACKNOWLEDGMENTS

THE investigations here reported were made possible by a grant provided by the Nuffield Foundation, at the request of Professor Sir Alexander Ewing, Director of the Department of Audiology and Education of the Deaf in the University of Manchester. Thanks are due to Sir Alexander Ewing for his assistance in the planning and carrying out of the research, and to the Nuffield Foundation for their financial assistance.

The co-operation of the Principal School Medical Officer for Cheshire is gratefully recorded. In all cases the utmost kindness and interest was shown by Head and Assistant teachers of schools in the County of Cheshire visited during the survey.

Thanks are also due to Mr. K. Harrison who carried out the E.N.T. examinations of many of the children included in the survey, and to Mr. H. Phillipson, Education Officer for the County Borough of Warrington, who kindly made facilities available for a pilot survey.

Much valuable advice was gained from discussions with members of the staff of the Department of Audiology and Education of the Deaf. Thanks are also due to Dr. H. Owrid, Mr. D. Sanders and Mr. G. Campbell, of the Department, who undertook the audiometric testing of children studied in the survey.

# CONTENTS

FOREWORD                                                              *page* v

ACKNOWLEDGMENTS                                                        vii

I.    INTRODUCTION                                                     I

II.   THE INCIDENCE OF IMPAIRED HEARING                                16

III.  FINDINGS FOR THE MAIN RESEARCH GROUP                            27

IV.   SPEECH DEVELOPMENT AND VERBAL ABILITY                           47

V.    THE USE OF HEARING AIDS                                         58

VI.   EMOTIONAL STABILITY AND SOCIAL ADJUSTMENT                       64

VII.  THE SCHOOLS AND CHILDREN WITH IMPAIRED HEARING                  78

VIII. SPECIAL PROVISIONS                                              85

IX.   CHESHIRE COUNTY CHILDREN IN SPECIAL SCHOOLS FOR
      THE DEAF AND PARTIALLY DEAF                                     95

X.    PLANNING EDUCATIONAL PROVISION                                  109

      BIBLIOGRAPHY                                                    117

      INDEX                                                           119

# CHAPTER I

## INTRODUCTION

INCREASING emphasis continues to be placed on the problems of the handicapped child by those concerned with the welfare and education of our children. In the field of hearing impairment, great technical advances, and significant changes in point of view as to educational provision, have taken place in the years since the war. The study here reported has dealt principally with children in ordinary primary and secondary schools handicapped by impaired hearing, and with the various provisions which are being made or could be made for them. Interest in this problem has been aroused, not only because of a desire to know more about the number and the condition of children with impaired hearing already attending ordinary schools, but also because of the trend towards greater integration of handicapped and unhandicapped children during their education. The matter is an extremely complex one in which both medical and educational specialists are involved, and there is no doubt that a great deal still remains to be done for children with impaired hearing in ordinary schools under the general headings of ascertainment, diagnosis, treatment, education and supervision. It is hoped that this book will help to add a small amount to our knowledge in each of these directions.

The 1956 Report of the Scottish Council for Research in Education[1] concerning the individual audiometric testing of 4,000 children of 12 years of age in Fife, states:

> There is very little evidence, however, on the degree of retardation in English and Arithmetic to be expected among pupils with minor defects of hearing, i.e. those pupils who continue to attend ordinary schools and whose defect is not sufficiently serious for them to require special educational treatment in schools for the deaf.

[1] *Hearing Defects of School Children*, Scottish Council for Research in Education.

1

The principal purpose of this study has been to obtain detailed information with regard to the educational attainments and the social adjustment of a group of children with impaired hearing attending ordinary schools. As will be seen later, such a group consists not only of those with minor defects of hearing but includes children who can remain with advantage in an ordinary school and those who might well, under present arrangements, be receiving special educational treatment but, for various reasons, have continued in an ordinary school.

A detailed audiological investigation was made in the case of each child. This provided information as to the type and degree of hearing impairment to be found amongst children in ordinary schools, and made possible an estimate of the relationship between certain types and patterns of hearing impairment and educational and social progress.

There has been a marked increase in recent years in the number of children attending ordinary schools who have been issued with hearing aids. An attempt was therefore made to consider various problems connected with their use, and to determine the extent to which hearing aids are of benefit to children in ordinary schools.

The opportunity was also taken to compare the findings for children with impaired hearing attending ordinary schools, with the audiological histories and educational attainments of children at present being educated in special schools for the deaf and partially deaf.

At the same time, methods of ascertainment, diagnosis and supervision (especially by peripatetic teachers of the deaf) were studied.

The findings in connection with the detailed study of a group of children with impaired hearing in ordinary schools have been derived from data obtained during personal visits to children attending ordinary schools in the county of Cheshire. Many discussions were held with medical, clinical and educational personnel working in the field, and personal visits were made to a number of units for the partially deaf and to schools for the deaf and partially deaf. In addition as much of the relevant literature as possible was studied.

Following the Report of the 1938 Committee of Inquiry into problems relating to 'Children with Defective Hearing' [1] (hereinafter referred to as the 1938 Report) the Board of Education endorsed the recommendation:

that routine group testing of all children in ordinary schools should be the basis of any scheme for the ascertainment and treatment of children with defective hearing.

However the 1939–45 war prevented many local authorities from giving effect to this recommendation and, although much has been done by certain authorities since the war, time has shown that the recommendation was an ambitious one. Audiometric testing, whether group or individual, of all children in ordinary schools is far from complete and there continues to be considerable doubt as to the number of children with defective hearing attending ordinary schools. Therefore a further aim of this study was to obtain a more precise estimate of the general incidence of hearing impairment amongst ordinary school children both from the evidence obtained in the Cheshire study and by obtaining returns to a questionnaire sent to certain local authorities. Details were requested of children with significant hearing impairment known to be attending ordinary schools and of the numbers issued with hearing aids. Information was sought as to the number of children attending special schools for the deaf and partially deaf and other types of special school; the use made of units for the partially deaf and peripatetic teachers, and the extent to which routine audiometric testing and screening procedures were being used. Returns of this nature do not usually include details of children attending private schools and an additional questionnaire was sent to private schools in the county of Cheshire requesting information concerning children with impaired hearing or with hearing aids, who might be attending such schools.

---

[1] Report of the Committee of Inquiry into Problems Relating to Children with Defective Hearing, H.M.S.O., 1938.

*Plan of Research and Selection of the Research Group*

The first stage of the study involved a pilot survey carried out in the County Borough of Warrington. A number of children who had been referred for testing of hearing to the Department of Education of the Deaf, University of Manchester, and who were attending ordinary schools in Warrington, were visited in their schools. Discussions were held with parents, head and assistant teachers and with the Director of Education. This pilot survey made it possible to estimate the work required in making school visits, and helped in the selection of tests and the preparation of suitable record forms. Moreover it confirmed the view that a programme of personal visits to the schools attended by children with impaired hearing should be an essential part of the main survey.

Facilities having been kindly made available to undertake school visiting in the county of Cheshire, preparations were then made to assemble a group of children with impaired hearing attending primary, secondary and private schools in the county. The total school population of the area (excluding county boroughs) is about 120,000. At the commencement of the survey no special provision was provided in Cheshire in the form of units for the partially deaf or peripatetic teachers of the deaf. Two peripatetic teachers of the deaf were, however, appointed shortly before the field work was completed.

It was not known at the outset how many children there were likely to be with impaired hearing attending ordinary schools, nor how many could be visited in the time available (i.e. approximately one year for field work and a further year for initial planning, visits to units for the partially deaf and special schools, and the writing of this report). Ascertainment was proceeding whilst the survey was taking place, at part-time consultant audiology clinics held at a number of centres in Cheshire to which children with suspected hearing impairment are referred. The research group was built up from children in the county already known to school medical officers to have significant hearing impairment, or children who were referred for diagnosis, or otherwise discovered, as the survey proceeded. No attempt was made to ascertain children by means of audiometric testing of selected age groups. Audiometric testing of whole age groups is not at present routine practice in the county.

It was decided to limit the scope of inquiry in the present survey to a detailed study of children attending ordinary schools with an average hearing impairment over 30 decibels (db.) in the better ear, whether or not they had been issued with hearing aids. The average hearing impairment was derived from summing and dividing by four the hearing loss in the better ear for pure tones[1] at the frequencies 500, 1,000, 2,000 and 4,000 cycles per second (c.p.s.). These frequencies were chosen because many studies have shown that there is a high correlation between the average loss of hearing for pure tones at these frequencies and the average loss of hearing for the principal sounds of speech. For this reason children with an average hearing impairment of less than 30 db. in the better ear over the frequencies 500 c.p.s. to 4,000 c.p.s. were excluded from the programme of personal school visits. Some such decision had to be made in order to ensure that the children forming the main research group were those with a hearing impairment likely to be the most significant factor in their educational and social progress. Whilst it is difficult to draw a dividing line in this way, the choice of 30 db. as the criterion in judging the border-line of significant hearing impairment is supported by the fact that a hearing aid would not generally be recommended for a child with an average hearing impairment in the better ear of less than 30 db. Children with an average hearing impairment of less than 30 db. were considered to fall into the Grade I classification as set out in the 1938 Report, i.e. 'Children with defective hearing who can, nevertheless, without special arrangements of any kind, obtain proper benefit from the education provided in an ordinary school.'

Considerable work was involved in discovering the names of suitable children to be included in the study, and in bringing

---

[1] The pure tone as used in audiometry is a single frequency (the simplest form of sound). Most sounds in nature consist of complex tones, i.e. a number of frequencies existing simultaneously.

together the necessary information concerning their medical and educational records. The procedure was by no means as easy as might be supposed and it demonstrated the difficulties of ascertainment and of obtaining full central records of children with impaired hearing. There is no doubt that the preparation of such records provides a complex task for school medical authorities, but it is not possible to provide medical and educational treatment unless there is a thorough knowledge of how many children and which children require treatment. A major effort is being made towards full ascertainment in Cheshire by means of referral of suspected cases of hearing impairment by school medical officers, and their examination at the consultant audiology clinics in the county.[1] But at the time the present study commenced, there were many undiagnosed cases of impaired hearing amongst the ordinary school population of the county, and the number of children known to have impaired hearing gradually increases as the intensive ascertainment programme continues. It is a matter of surprise to many people that ascertainment of a handicap, of which we are by no means unaware, can be incomplete. The layman might well be excused for supposing that the responsible authorities in all areas would be in a position to know more than they do of the children with hearing impairment or, for that matter, with any defect likely to be a handicap in their education. The medical staff available, the size of the area and of the school population are factors which make the difficulties greater in some areas than in others and there are, of course, factors inherent in the nature of hearing impairment in particular, which pose special problems to be discussed in the body of this report. However, there is also a lack of knowledge about the subject, its complexity and its extent which is certainly larger than many authorities suppose.

It was decided, in the first place, to obtain a list of children attending ordinary schools known by the school medical authorities in Cheshire to have been issued with hearing aids. Some of the

---

[1] These clinics are conducted either by Professor Sir Alexander Ewing or Dr. I. G. Taylor of the Department of Audiology and Education of the Deaf, University of Manchester, in co-operation with assistant medical officers of the Health Department, Cheshire County Council.

children so named had either left school or left the district since the list was prepared, or had been transferred to special schools for the partially deaf, but sufficient names were available for school visiting to commence. For various reasons, to be discussed in the section of the report dealing with hearing aids, information concerning the issue of a hearing aid does not aways reach the school medical authorities so that this list was by no means complete.

Further names of children either issued with hearing aids, or with significant hearing impairment but not issued with hearing aids, were obtained from the following sources:

Examination of case notes of children referred for testing of hearing at the Department of Audiology and Education of the Deaf, University of Manchester.

Examination of records of children referred for testing of hearing at the Regional Audiology Clinics in Cheshire.

Letters of inquiry to E.N.T. Departments of hospitals serving the area.

Examination of case records of children referred for testing of hearing by school medical officers during the course of the survey.

Letters of inquiry to private schools in the county.

Information obtained from head teachers, teachers and parents with whom discussions were held in the course of the survey.

Eventually a group of 68 children with average hearing impairment of over 30 db. in the better ear was assembled. This number does not, of course, constitute all the children in Cheshire known to fall into this category, but only those for whom full records were obtainable and who were known at the time the survey was in progress.

Since it is unusual to find more than one or two children with impaired hearing in the same school, the area to be covered was considerable and, in some cases, a school visit to see one child could involve a round journey of 120 miles. The procedures of finding suitable children and of school visiting continued from February 1959 to the end of March 1960.

The following information was sought in the case of each child:

*Audiological.* Results of hearing tests for both bone and air conduction, an evaluation of the type and pattern of deafness, results of speech audiometry and information as to the age of onset of deafness.

*Medical.* Reports of E.N.T. consultants, medical history of the child and parents, probable cause of deafness, medical or surgical treatment given.

*Hearing Aids.* Type of hearing aid, date issued and place of issue. Attitude of the children towards their hearing aids. Details of any training in the use of an aid. Extent to which aids were used in school and at home. Maintenance of hearing aids.

*Speech Development.* Results of speech tests given in the schools (monitored by means of a sound level indicator) under classroom conditions, and in a quiet room in the school. An estimate of the intelligibility of the child's speech made by teachers and by the investigator. A measure of ability in the comprehension of spoken language. The material used for the monitored speech tests consisted of the M.J. word lists designed in, and used by, the Department of Audiology and Education of the Deaf at Manchester University.

*Educational.* An Arithmetic Age and Reading Age was obtained using the Schonell Essential Arithmetic Test and the Schonell Graded Word Reading Test. Results were also available in most cases of standardised tests used in Cheshire at various stages, i.e. Burt Reading Test, Southend Arithmetic Attainment Test and Moray House Arithmetic Tests. The Raven's Matrices Test (1938 version) was given individually by the investigator to obtain a measure of non-verbal intellectual ability. Results of verbal tests of intelligence set by teachers were also available in some cases. In addition, estimates were obtained from teachers as to the general school progress of the children.

*Personal/Social.* Information was obtained regarding these factors by means of questionnaire to teachers, discussions with parents and personal observation. The questionnaire sought details of emotional disorders (withdrawal, day-dreaming, tics, be-

haviour problems, obsessional behaviour), social maturity, relationships with other children and with adults.

In addition the attitudes of other children, teachers and parents
towards the child with impaired hearing was studied.

The procedure adopted in most cases was, in the first place, a
discussion with the head teacher and the completion as far as
possible of the standard record form used in the study. Speech
audiometry and individual tests of intelligence and attainment
were then given to the child. Finally speech tests were given under
classroom conditions, and a discussion was held with the class
teacher or teachers having close knowledge of the child. If parents
were able to be present, a discussion was held with them in the
schools or, if this was not possible, the parents were seen in their
homes.

*Previous Inquiries*

It is only possible in this summary to mention recent studies
specifically concerned with impaired hearing amongst ordinary
school children, but its significance as a factor in educational
retardation has often been pointed out in more general surveys of
backwardness (notably by Burt and Schonell).

The first major report dealing with the problem of hearing
impairment amongst ordinary school children was the 1938
Report when the findings and views of the leading experts of the
day were obtained.[1] This report is perhaps best known for its
classification of children with defective hearing into educational
grades. The definition of Grade I children in the 1938 Report has
been referred to above. Grade II was sub-divided into Grade IIA,
'children who can make satsifactory progress in ordinary classes
in ordinary schools provided they are given some help, whether
by way of favourable position in class, by individual hearing aids,
or by tuition in lipreading', and Grade IIB, 'children who fail to
make satisfactory progress in ordinary schools'. Grade III consisted of children without naturally acquired speech requiring
special education, but for the most part these children were outside

[1] Report of the Committee of Inquiry into Problems Relating to Children
with Defective Hearing.

the scope of the inquiry. On this basis the majority of the children studied in the present survey would be those classified as Grade IIA. However, the exact terminology to be used in the classification of children with defective hearing has continued to present problems and to be a matter of controversy. In this report it is not proposed to make use of the terms 'deaf' or 'partially deaf' for the children studied in this survey, but to refer only to the general term of 'impaired hearing'. This is because, to the layman, the term 'deaf' implies a child without hearing for any sounds, which is a relatively rare condition even amongst children with defective hearing as a whole, and certainly does not apply to any of the children studied in this survey. The 1938 Report would have preferred to see the term 'partially deaf' discontinued but, despite the fact that it is an inexact and rather anomalous term, it is still in common use. But the principle of classification on an educational basis, rather than on the grounds of hearing loss or speech development alone, has for long been accepted as a sound one. The findings of the present study would tend to suggest that, in many cases, the educational basis of classification could be given even more weight than it has been since the 1938 Report in determining placement. That is to say that certain children can manage in the ordinary school with severer hearing impairment than is generally considered suitable at present.

So far as causation of deafness is concerned the 1938 Report has, quite naturally, been out-dated by subsequent findings. Generally the Report only considered conditions leading to conductive deafness, i.e. suppurative otitis media, catarrhal otitis media, bad environmental conditions and poor diet; no distinction was made between conductive and perceptive deafness. Whilst there is therefore no information as to the extent of perceptive deafness amongst ordinary school children at the time the 1938 Report was compiled, it is clear from the findings of the present survey that the majority of such children with significant hearing impairment (i.e. over 30 db. in the better ear) have perceptive deafness.[1] It is not suggested for one moment, even allowing for new forms of medical treatment, that conductive deafness does not continue to

[1] See Table 7, p. 39.

present a difficult problem, but it is recommended that a clearer distinction be made between conductive and perceptive deafness. Conductive deafness, i.e. where the organ of hearing is normal but there is a mal-development or acquired disorder of the sound-conducting part of the auditory apparatus, differs from perceptive deafness in that it is less severe; much more common in cases of impaired hearing as a whole; owing to its acquired nature and the site of the disorders it presents less of a problem in speech development and discrimination and, most important, hearing may be restored to within normal limits by appropriate medical or surgical treatment. On the other hand perceptive deafness, i.e. when the outer and middle ear is normal but there is damage to the inner ear or the auditory nerve, is more severe and, being at present not amenable to medical treatment, is a permanent handicap; moreover it nearly always results in defective speech development, and the difficulties in speech discrimination are much greater. There are other distinctions, connected with the pattern of hearing loss and the use of hearing aids, but the above represents the principal differences between the two types of deafness. In conductive deafness the medical problem is greater than the educational, whilst in perceptive deafness educational and social considerations take precedence over the medical.

The 1938 Report stressed the benefits likely to be obtained from the use of individual hearing aids and this has been confirmed by subsequent experience. The formation of classes attached to ordinary schools was not recommended, although this has since become common practice and seems to be expanding rapidly.

In 1948 Sheridan's work on defective speech in school children made considerable reference to the effects of hearing impairment on speech development.[1] Besides charting the nature of the speech of a hundred children with impaired hearing, information was also obtained about their educational attainments. Amongst this group there were a number with relatively slight impairment, and again no clear distinction was made between conductive and perceptive deafness. However, Sheridan was able to give valuable information as to the type of speech defect found amongst the children

[1] Sheridan, M. D., *The Child's Hearing for Speech.*

with high tone hearing loss which, though quite distinct from other forms of speech defect, is still likely to be mistakenly attributed to handicaps other than deafness. So far as educational attainments were concerned, Sheridan found that the scores of her subjects for all the linguistic subjects were well below average. It is interesting to note that such a relatively short time ago the use of individual hearing aids was most uncommon, and Sheridan states 'several older children of good intelligence were provided with hearing aids with disappointing results and it was not found possible to provide hearing aids for younger children since they cannot learn to adjust them with sufficient care and precision'. Sheridan's study was most important because it so clearly set out the relationship between speech and hearing which, as the present investigation shows, is still not fully appreciated either in the recognition of the specific speech defects associated with hearing impairment, or in the full acceptance of the fact that the child with defective hearing and speech has, in effect, a dual handicap of a very serious nature.

The 1950 Report of the Advisory Council on Education in Scotland, unlike the 1938 Report, dealt with the problems of all grades of hearing defect but refers in some detail to the particular problems of children able to manage in an ordinary school.[1] The report stressed the need for early ascertainment of deafness and pointed out that the incidence of all forms of deafness save the most gross is not known with accuracy. The Council suggested the need for an audiometric and educational survey of large numbers of children with impaired hearing, and recommended that in any such survey 'some standardised measure should be made of primary school attainment in speech and reading'. Causation of deafness was mainly considered under the headings of the congenital and adventitious, but again no distinction was made between conductive and perceptive deafness. It is interesting to note that at this date the report states: 'Hearing aids have seldom been provided in Scotland for Grade IIA children' (i.e. children able to manage in an ordinary school). Instruction in lipreading was

[1] *Pupils who are Defective in Hearing*, Report of the Advisory Council on Education in Scotland.

recommended for such children, but the setting up of classes for lipreading as such has largely been discontinued at present in England and Wales, although they are still used in Scotland.

In fulfilment of the recommendation made in the above-mentioned report, an audiometric and educational survey was carried out in Fife by the Scottish Council for Research in Education and the results were published in 1956.[1] In all, 4,170 children of 12 years of age were given audiometric tests and their results in the Intelligence, English and Arithmetic papers of the Secondary school transfer examination were obtained. 325 children were found to have a defect of hearing according to the criteria of defect adopted (i.e. failure at 10 db. on any frequency from 250 to 4,000 c.p.s. in a threshold test by pure-tone audiometer), but only 28 had hearing impairment of over 30 db. in the better ear and eight of these were attending special schools. So that the survey dealt with only 20 children attending ordinary schools with an impairment similar to that judged as significant in the present study. It is therefore not possible to put a great deal of weight on the findings for such a small group, but it was noted that, of this group, only 50 per cent were already known to their teachers to have a hearing defect. The findings of the present study confirm that it is not uncommon for children with hearing impairment over 30 db. to be unrecognised as such by their teachers. As to social development, the evidence was not sufficient to associate any particular type of unusual behaviour with defective hearing, whereas this study reveals a definite pattern of behaviour often found in children with impaired hearing. The Fife survey also showed that when the audiological records of the 325 children with defective hearing were examined, 217 of them were found to have one normal ear, and that all of these children were in the category of hearing impairment below 30 db. It is thus likely that the decision in the present survey not to include children with hearing impairment below 30 db. in the detailed programme of personal visits was a necessary one if the effect of significant hearing impairment was to be studied.

[1] *Hearing Defects of School Children*, Scottish Council for Research in Education.

In Australia, from 1947 to 1955, Brereton studied a group of 90 children with hearing impairment mainly caused by maternal rubella.[1] Most of this group attended special schools or classes, but 24 who had an appreciable experience in a normal school were compared with a similar number who were without experience in a normal school—the groups being matched for hearing loss (average loss for both groups being between 50 and 60 db.) and intelligence. Brereton records that 'the most marked difference between the achievement of children attending and not attending normal school occurred in clarity of speech, in skill in repeating sentences and in tests of understanding spoken language'. None of the 24 children who did not have experience in a normal school reached at age $11\frac{1}{2}$ the mean score in tests of clarity of speech of those who did. Brereton concludes: 'Children with experience in ordinary schools are likely to speak more clearly and to accept a longer pattern of language as a unit than children attending special schools.' She states further: 'The increase in efficiency in speech of children who attend ordinary schools is not merely a reflection of the sounds they hear. It probably occurs because the rhythmic patterns of normal speech are encountered in situations which give meaning to the patterns as a whole.' The latter applied despite the fact that, as Brereton states, 'a normal classroom does not seem a particularly good place for actually hearing words, nor a place likely to provide frequent experience of listening to language that can be readily understood'. The findings of the present study support Brereton's conclusions; it has not been found that the admittedly poor acoustic conditions existing in many of the schools visited, outweigh the advantages to be obtained in the ordinary school environment in developing intelligible and fluent speech. On the other hand Brereton also found retardation, sometimes by as much as four years, in tests of skill in reading and in knowledge of numbers amongst her group of children in ordinary schools. Similarly the present study has shown marked educational retardation amongst many of the group of children with hearing impairment over 30 db. and these facts have to be set against the findings of improved facility in speech and language.

[1] Brereton, B. Le Gay, *The Schooling of Children with Impaired Hearing*.

In 1959 Ling reported the study of 69 children with defects of hearing in the Borough of Reading.[1] 42 of the children attended ordinary schools but the majority of them had an average hearing impairment under 25 db. Only 15 of the ordinary school group had average hearing impairment between 26 and 65 db. Even so the mean retardation for the group was sixteen months in Mechanical Arithmetic and fifteen months in Reading. The mean intelligence for the group was reported as being above the average. This study would seem to indicate that, even when hearing impairment is relatively slight, educational retardation may result. However, factors other than hearing impairment may have contributed to the retardation of those children with hearing impairment under 25 db. It would require a large and carefully controlled study to determine with certainty the effect of slight hearing impairment on educational attainments.

Previous inquiries show that studies of children with impaired hearing attending ordinary schools have generally involved small numbers. In view of the relatively low incidence of hearing impairment it is necessary to cover a large area, or to bring together a great number of children for screen testing, if a research group of any size is to be produced. Even so, in the case of the Fife survey, when 4,170 children were screen tested, only a small number of children with significant hearing impairment in ordinary schools was discovered. The method adopted in the present study, i.e. the study of children referred for suspected deafness from a large area, has not produced an exceptionally large group of children suitable by reason of age and hearing impairment for detailed study. However, the number of children available has been greater than in previous studies and it is hoped that a small step forward in our knowledge of their problems has been made possible.

[1] Ling, D., 'The Education and General Background of Children with Defective Hearing in Reading', Cambridge Institute of Education Library, 1959.

# CHAPTER II

## THE INCIDENCE OF IMPAIRED HEARING

IN the course of this study information was obtained from certain local authorities as to the number of children being sent to special schools for the deaf and partially deaf, the number issued with hearing aids and attending ordinary schools or other types of special school, and the number considered to have significant hearing impairment in ordinary schools but not issued with hearing aids. Questionnaries were sent to twenty-four local education authorities and twenty replies were received from eight county boroughs and twelve county councils; eleven returns were from urban areas and nine from rural areas. The total school population for all the areas is about $2\frac{3}{4}$ million. The figures received are discussed below in relation to a number of previous estimates of incidence and to the evidence obtained in Cheshire.

### 1. *Children attending Special Schools for the Deaf and Partially Deaf*

The 1938 Report gave an estimate of 0·7 to 1·0 per 1,000 school children in their Grade III classification, i.e. children requiring education in a school for the deaf, and 0·5 per 1,000 in their Grade IIB classification, i.e. children requiring education in schools for the partially deaf.

In the Ministry of Education Pamphlet No. 5 the incidence of deaf pupils is given as 1·0 per 1,000 and the incidence of partially deaf pupils as 1·0 per 1,000 and upwards.[1]

In 1950 the Advisory Council on Education in Scotland suggested a revision of the estimates in the 1938 Report for Grade III to 0·7 per 1,000 and for Grade IIB to 0·5 to 1·0 per 1,000.[2] The Report of the Scottish Council for Research in Education, discussing an audiometric survey of 4,000 children of 12 years of age

---

[1] *Special Educational Treatment*, Ministry of Education Pamphlet No. 5.
[2] *Pupils who are defective in Hearing.*

in Fife, considered the 1938 Report estimate for Grade III to be on the low side.[1]

The figures obtained in the present survey for children attending schools for the deaf and the partially deaf are set out in Table 1. The returns show a degree of variation in incidence ranging from 0·38 to 1·34 per 1,000 of the total school population. The mean for rural areas is 0·63 and for urban areas 0·80, with an overall mean

TABLE I

Numbers of Children at Special Schools for the Deaf and Partially Deaf in 20 Local Authorities

|  | Total School Population 1,000's | Children at Schools for Deaf | Children at Schools for Partially Deaf | Incidence per 1,000 |
|---|---|---|---|---|
| COUNTY COUNCILS |  |  |  |  |
| I | 286 | 96 | 94 | 0·66 |
| II | 162 | 100 | 29 | 0·80 |
| III | 19 | 7 | 3 | 0·53 |
| IV | 122 | 42 | 47 | 0·73 |
| V | 66 | 23 | 21 | 0·67 |
| VI | 102 | 46 | 11 | 0·56 |
| VII | 300 | 172 | 88 | 0·87 |
| VIII | 37 | 11 | 3 | 0·38 |
| IX | 74 | 26 | 12 | 0·51 |
| X | 436 | 292 | 50 | 0·78 |
| XI | 120 | 56 | 54 | 0·91 |
| XII | 322 | 155 | 101 | 0·80 |
| COUNTY BOROUGHS |  |  |  |  |
| I | 52 | 28 | 11 | 0·75 |
| II | 134 | 107 | 72 | 1·34 |
| III | 116 | 79 | 1 | 0·69 |
| IV | 42 | 38 | 9 | 1·11 |
| V | 42 | 18 | 4 | 0·52 |
| VI | 180 | 202 |  | 1·21 |
| VII | 28 | 18 | Nil | 0·64 |
| VIII | 178 | 49 | 61 | 0·62 |

of 0·73 per 1,000. It has generally been accepted on the basis of previous estimates that an incidence of 1·0 per 1,000 for deaf children and 0·05 for partially deaf children is a reasonable estimate

[1] *Hearing Defects of School Children*, S.C.E.D.

of the number of children likely to be in need of special schooling. The incidence of children being sent to schools for the deaf and partially deaf in the present returns (i.e. 0·73 per 1,000) is thus lower than previous estimates. However it agrees closely with the actual numbers of children on roll in the special schools compared with the total school population of England and Wales,[1] i.e. 4,898 as against 6,839,518, giving an incidence of 0·75 per 1,000. Most of these children would have perceptive deafness and it is interesting to compare this last estimate with that of Johnsen who, from the results of a survey of 109,000 school children in Denmark, estimated the incidence of bilateral perceptive deafness to be 0·64 per 1,000 for children in special schools.[2] But there are also deaf and partially deaf children in other types of special school (0·1 per 1,000, for example, in special schools in the London County Council area), in private schools for the deaf, or remaining in ordinary schools though recommended for special school placement. Allowing for such children, an estimate of 1 per 1,000 school children considered at the present time to be in need of special schooling, either in schools for the deaf or partially deaf, must be very nearly correct.

Further examination of the returns in the present survey, shows that variations from the mean for the number of children being sent to special schools are found in areas providing accommodation for partially deaf children in units attached to ordinary schools. There were eight such authorities amongst those sending returns and, excluding them, the mean figure for deaf and partially deaf children sent to special schools increases from 0·73 to 0·88 per 1,000. Such variations are, of course, more evident in the numbers of children sent to schools for the partially deaf. Considering the figures for children sent to schools for the partially deaf separately, the range is from nil (in one area) to 0·23 per 1,000, with a mean of 0·13 per 1,000. In areas without units for the partially deaf attached to ordinary schools a mean figure of 0·29 per

[1] *The Health of the School Child*, Report of the Chief Medical Officer of the Ministry of Education for the years 1956 and 1957.
[2] Johnsen, Steen, 'Incidence and Correlation between Aetiology and Audiometric Pattern', *Journal of Laryngology and Otology*, 1957.

1,000 school children are being sent to schools for the partially deaf, with a range from 0·08 to 0·54 per 1,000. It is interesting to note that the area without special units sending the smallest number of children to schools for the partially deaf, has the highest number of children issued with hearing aids and attending ordinary schools. The increase in numbers of children in ordinary schools being issued with hearing aids, and in the number of units for partially deaf children attached to ordinary schools, would seem to indicate a possible falling off in the number of children likely to be sent to schools for the partially deaf in the future.

## 2. Children attending other types of Special School

In order to estimate the number of children with impaired hearing attending special schools other than those for the deaf and partially deaf, a questionnaire was sent to eighteen of the local authorities participating in the survey of incidence. Replies were received from sixteen of these authorities (total school population 2,129,000) and the data obtained is discussed below.

The authorities were asked to state the number of children at other types of special school who had been issued with hearing aids. Information was also sought concerning the number of children issued with hearing aids attending occupation centres for the ineducable, and the number of children sent to schools for the deaf and partially deaf and subsequently found to be ineducable.

The returns for children issued with hearing aids attending special schools other than those for the deaf and partially deaf are set out in Table 1. It can be seen from Table 1 that the largest numbers of children issued with hearing aids are attending schools for E.S.N., physically handicapped and delicate children, in that order. The total number of children attending other types of special school is as follows: E.S.N. children, 30,656; delicate, 11,000; physically handicapped, 6,779; partially sighted, 1,819; maladjusted, 1,642, and blind, 1,279.[1] The number of children issued with hearing aids at these schools is closely related to the total numbers of children attending them. The reason for the

[1] *Education in 1959*, H.M.S.O., 1960.

relatively higher number of children issued with hearing aids in schools for the physically handicapped than in schools for delicate children, is probably due to the high incidence of hearing impairment amongst children suffering from cerebral palsy.[1] It is evident that there are an appreciable number of children with

TABLE I

Numbers of Children issued with Hearing Aids attending Special Schools other than those for the Deaf and Partially Deaf in 16 Areas

| | Total School Population 1,000's | (1) | (2) | (3) | (4) | (5) | (6) | Totals |
|---|---|---|---|---|---|---|---|---|
| COUNTY COUNCILS | | | | | | | | |
| 1 | 110 | 0 | 1 | 1 | 3 | 0 | 0 | 5 |
| 2 | 66 | 0 | 0 | 1 | 1 | 0 | 0 | 2 |
| 3 | 19 | 0 | 1 | 1 | 0 | 0 | 0 | 2 |
| 4 | 37 | 0 | 0 | 1 | 2 | 0 | 0 | 3 |
| 5 | 163 | 0 | 0 | 2 | 0 | 0 | 1 | 3 |
| 6 | 287 | 0 | 2 | 12 | 7 | 1 | 3 | 25 |
| 7 | 128 | 0 | 0 | 6 | 3 | 0 | 0 | 9 |
| 8 | 300 | 2 | 0 | 13 | 5 | 1 | 3 | 24 |
| 9 | 433 | 2 | 3 | 22 | 13 | 1 | 4 | 45 |
| COUNTY BOROUGHS | | | | | | | | |
| 1 | 27 | 0 | 0 | 6 | 0 | 0 | 2 | 8 |
| 2 | 132 | 1 | 0 | 13 | 3 | 0 | 1 | 18 |
| 3 | 44 | 0 | 0 | 4 | 0 | 0 | 1 | 5 |
| 4 | 114 | 0 | 0 | 3 | 3 | 1 | 0 | 7 |
| 5 | 52 | 0 | 0 | 3 | 1 | 1 | 0 | 5 |
| 6 | 43 | 1 | 0 | 4 | 1 | 1 | 2 | 9 |
| 7 | 184 | 0 | 1 | 5 | 3 | 0 | 4 | 13 |
| Totals | | 6 | 8 | 97 | 45 | 6 | 21 | 183 |

KEY

*Type of Special School:* (1) Blind; (2) Partially Sighted; (3) Educationally Subnormal; (4) Physically Handicapped; (5) Maladjusted; (6) Delicate.

[1] For notes on the incidence of hearing impairment amongst cerebral palsied children, see *Health of the School Child*, 1956–7 (p. 119).

impaired hearing in other types of special school, and sufficient to require specialist interest in their particular problems and welfare.

Twenty-three children attending occupation centres in thirteen of the authorities had been issued with hearing aids. Fourteen of the authorities gave returns of the number of children sent to schools for the deaf and since found ineducable. In seven of these authorities there were no such children, and for the remaining seven authorities the total number of such children over the last three years was 21.

### 3. *Children attending Ordinary Schools*

The number of children with impaired hearing able to manage in an ordinary school with some form of special help is by no means as easy to estimate. Previous estimates have been based on two main categories: (*a*) children able to manage in an ordinary school without help of any kind (the Grade I of the 1938 Report), and (*b*) children able to manage in an ordinary school with special help (the Grade IIA of the 1938 Report). These are very broad categories and do not allow for any distinction between perceptive and conductive deafness or between bilateral and unilateral deafness. The difference between perceptive and conductive deafness is so marked (see p. 11) that it is really necessary to consider the incidence of perceptive and conductive deafness separately. In the main it is likely that the children most in need of special help in the ordinary school will be those with perceptive deafness or mixed perceptive and conductive deafness.[1] The children with pure conductive hearing impairment, amongst whom there will be many with unilateral deafness, really represent a separate category. Johnsen, in the study mentioned above (p. 18), estimated an incidence of 2 per 1,000 children in Denmark suffering from bilateral perceptive deafness, i.e. excluding children being educated in the special schools. Most of the children requiring hearing aids fall into this category. Estimates made in American studies of children likely to benefit from the use of hearing aids in ordinary school, suggest a fair estimate of incidence for such children to

[1] See Table 7, p. 39.

be about 1·4 per 1,000.[1] In Reading, where there has been very careful ascertainment, there were, in 1958, 2·0 per 1,000 children attending ordinary schools who had been issued with hearing aids.[2] The highest incidence for this category obtained in the present returns was 1·4 per 1,000 school children. The complete figures for children issued with hearing aids attending ordinary schools obtained in the present survey are set out in Table 2. The mean incidence for children issued with hearing aids for the twenty local authorities is 0·56 per 1,000 but the range is considerable, the lowest incidence being 0·23 and the highest 1·4 per 1,000. It has to be remembered, of course, that the issue of Medresco transistor hearing aids through the National Health Service has only been in operation since mid-1958. Nevertheless, the range in the incidence of children issued with hearing aids attending ordinary schools probably reflects the achievements in ascertainment in different areas, and the confidence shown in the value of hearing aids. It would seem reasonable to conclude that a figure of 2 per 1,000 school children is a fair estimate of the incidence of bilateral deafness, perceptive or mixed perceptive and conductive, sufficiently marked to require some form of special help (including the use of a hearing aid) but not severe enough to require special schooling.

As to the incidence of conductive hearing impairment amongst ordinary school children, this poses an even more difficult problem. The needs of children with perceptive hearing impairment are very great, but the problem here is primarily one of ascertainment and educational provision. Children with conductive hearing impairment, besides having educational difficulties, present a complex task for school medical officers in so far as ascertainment, diagnosis and treatment are concerned. It is hard to say which of these two groups present the greater or more urgent problem. In many ways, and particularly because of their greater number, the conductive category, in so far as diagnosis and medical treatment

[1] Siegenthaler, B. M., 'Use of Hearing Aids by Public School Children'.
Gardner, W., Report of Committee on Hard of Hearing Children, *Hearing News*, 1950.
[2] Report of the Principal School Medical Officer for Reading, 1958.

## TABLE 2

Numbers of Children issued with Hearing Aids attending Ordinary
Schools in 20 Areas

|  | Total School Population 1,000's | Children issued with Hearing Aids | Incidence per 1,000 |
|---|---|---|---|
| COUNTY COUNCILS |  |  |  |
| I | 286 | 154 | 0·54 |
| II | 162 | 77 | 0·48 |
| III | 19 | 9 | 0·47 |
| IV | 122 | 88 | 0·72 |
| V | 66 | 15 | 0·23 |
| VI | 102 | 49 | 0·48 |
| VII | 300 | 229 | 0·76 |
| VIII | 37 | 53 | 1·40 |
| IX | 74 | 72 | 0·97 |
| X | 436 | 183 | 0·43 |
| XI | 120 | 80 | 0·67 |
| XII | 322 | 140 | 0·43 |
| COUNTY BOROUGHS |  |  |  |
| I | 52 | 18 | 0·35 |
| II | 134 | 61 | 0·45 |
| III | 116 | 31 | 0·27 |
| IV | 42 | 17 | 0·40 |
| V | 42 | 32 | 0·76 |
| VI | 180 | 82 | 0·46 |
| VII | 28 | 12 | 0·43 |
| VIII | 178 | 87 | 0·49 |

are concerned, is the more involved. It is probable that most
children classified as Grade I under the recommendations of the
1938 Report (i.e. children able to manage in an ordinary school
without special help of any kind) would have a conductive or
mixed conductive and perceptive impairment of hearing. The
1938 Report estimated Grade I incidence to be in the region of 50
to 80 per 1,000 school children. The 1950 Report of the Advisory
Council on Education in Scotland agreed with this estimate.[1] In
the Fife survey, 73 per 1,000 children were said to fall into a

[1] Report of the Advisory Council on Education in Scotland.

c

category generally approximating to Grade I.[1] Whilst it has always been accepted that the incidence of conductive deafness is much greater than that of perceptive deafness, it is felt that the above estimates are misleading. Indeed it seems pointless to have a category of children who can manage without special help of any kind. What is required is an estimate of the incidence of conductive hearing impairment which is sufficiently marked to be an educational handicap or to require medical treatment. It is true that from seventy to ninety children might fail an initial screening test, especially if the test is given at a level of 10 db. but this number is considerably reduced after further and more detailed audiometric testing. Moreover, a large number of those children who still show a defect will have normal hearing in one ear. In Glasgow, where audiometric surveys have been carried out annually since 1949, and over 140,000 children screen tested, it has been shown that, whereas 90 per 1,000 children may be expected to fail a screening test at the 10 db. level, only 42 per 1,000 would still fail more detailed audiometric tests. 77 per cent of the children failing the second audiometric test would have a minor, often unilateral, hearing impairment, whilst 21·3 per cent would be expected to have a marked hearing impairment corresponding to the Grade II classification.[2] On the basis of these findings, the incidence of children with some hearing defect, often very slight and unilateral, might be estimated as 30 per 1,000. The incidence of marked hearing impairment, over and above the 2 per 1,000 already estimated as having bilateral perceptive hearing impairment, might be estimated at about 10 per 1,000, and it is suggested that the majority of these children would have a conductive hearing impairment.

In a county the size of Cheshire (school population about 120,000) the above estimates would represent a figure of about 240 children with bilateral perceptive hearing impairment, most of whom would probably benefit from the use of a hearing aid. The latest figures available show that some 90 children attending

[1] *Hearing Defects of School Children.*
[2] From data kindly provided by the Principal School Medical Officer for Glasgow.

ordinary schools in Cheshire have been issued with hearing aids. The experience obtained in the Regional Audiology Clinics in Chesire, i.e. the rate at which referrals are being made and the number of children being recommended to use a hearing aid, show that the number of children using hearing aids could be considerably increased, if not doubled. From the evidence available in Cheshire it is felt that the estimate of 2 per 1,000 children with marked bilateral perceptive impairment who do not require special schooling is a realistic one. In addition there might be 10 per 1,000 or 1,200 children with a marked conductive hearing impairment requiring either medical treatment or educational supervision or both. Besides these children one might expect to find in Cheshire a further 30 per 1,000 or 3,600 children with a sufficient degree of hearing impairment to warrant an otological examination, but of these many would have a slight and often unilateral hearing impairment.

The programme of ascertainment at present being carried out in Cheshire, i.e. the referral of children with suspected hearing impairment for examination at the Regional Audiology Clinics, has led to the discovery of a considerable number of children with impaired hearing. As it continues probably the bulk of those children with marked hearing impairment will eventually be ascertained. However, to make sure that all children with a hearing impairment sufficient to warrant an otological examination become known, routine screening procedures would have to be adopted for pre-school and school children. That this is so is shown by the fact that whilst there are 120 Cheshire children of school age now attending special schools for the deaf and partially deaf, only 38 pre-school children with hearing impairment have at present been ascertained, not all of whom will eventually require special schooling.

The return of information from private schools in Cheshire is incomplete as only twenty-nine replies were received to the sixty-four letters of inquiry sent. From these returns, and from details already known about children in private schools, the number of children with impaired hearing known to attend such schools is 15, 11 of whom have been issued with hearing aids. It is possible that schools not replying would, in any case, have given a nil return. However there must be, in the country as a whole, a considerable number of children with impaired hearing who attend private schools.

# CHAPTER III

# FINDINGS FOR THE MAIN RESEARCH GROUP

THE audiograms and medical records of about 150 children attending ordinary schools in Cheshire who had been referred for testing of hearing were examined. 90 of these children were visited in their schools and a group numbering 68 (31 girls and 37 boys) were included in the detailed study of children with a hearing impairment of over 30 db. in the better ear. The remainder of those visited were excluded, either because their average hearing impairment was below 30 db., or because for various reasons adequate audiological and educational testing was not possible. The main findings with regard to this group of 68 children with hearing impairment over 30 db. are given below.

## Ages and Type of School attended

The ages of the children ranged from 5 to 15 and the numbers for particular ages are given in Table 3. Table 4 shows the type of school attended. The various reasons why these children were attending ordinary schools are given in Table 5. It will be seen

TABLE 3

Chronological ages of 68 Children with Hearing Impairment over 30 db.

| Chronological Age | Number of Pupils | Chronological Age | Number of Pupils |
|---|---|---|---|
| 5·0– 5·11 | 3 | 11·0–11·11 | 12 |
| 6·0– 6·11 | 4 | 12·0–12·11 | 8 |
| 7·0– 7·11 | 7 | 13·0–13·11 | 8 |
| 8·0– 8·11 | 4 | 14·0–14·11 | 5 |
| 9·0– 9·11 | 10 | 15·0–15·11 | 2 |
| 10·0–10·11 | 5 | | |

TABLE 4

Type of School attended

| Type of School | Number of Pupils |
|---|---|
| Infant | 6 |
| Junior | 36 |
| Secondary Modern | 19 |
| Secondary Grammar | 2 |
| Private | 5 |

TABLE 5

Reasons for attendance at Ordinary School for the 68 Children
with an average Hearing Impairment of over 30 db.

| | Number of Pupils |
|---|---|
| Recommended as suitable | 25 |
| Late or delayed diagnosis | 6 |
| Awaiting decision as to placement | 2 |
| Refused special school place | 5 |
| Awaiting special school place | 10 |
| Trial period in ordinary school | 7 |
| Transferred from special school | 1 |
| No specific recommendation made | 12 |

from Table 5 that only 37 per cent of the group were definitely recommended as likely to benefit from ordinary schooling, and that the majority were in ordinary schools either because no special recommendation had been made as to their education, or because of delays in diagnosis and placement. It is not the case that the group was made up entirely of children who had been correctly placed in ordinary schools after due consideration of their needs. If it were possible and practicable for every case to be decided before the age of 5 years, save those where onset of deafness is after the age of 5, this situation could probably have been achieved. In practice, however, diagnosis is often not made until much later than this and the procedure involved in arriving at a decision as to placement may often be a long drawn out one. Even so, the recommendations made are not always carried out, as parents sometimes refuse to co-operate. Out of the 42 children in the group whose ages at first referral were known, only nine had been referred before the age of 5 years. Nine were referred after the age of 11, and the remainder at various ages between 5 and 11 years. From these figures the need for earlier ascertainment and decisions as to placement is clearly indicated.

An example of a late decision in placement is given below:

CASE T.J. Boy. Age 10·7. Primary School.

Referred by the County E.N.T. Consultant for investigation of hearing at age 9·8. Seen three months later for audiological and otological examination when special education in a school for partially deaf children was recommended. At the time of this examination his mother said that deafness had been noticed at about 3 years of age. At age 10·3 it was suggested by the School Medical authorities that, owing to the lengthy waiting list for admission to a school for the partially deaf, he might be better placed in a school for pupils with dual handicaps—in his case deafness and suspected mental retardation. However, at the same age, he was given an intelligence test by the present investigator which showed him to be of average mental ability. At age 10·7 he was visited in school during the course of the study here reported: his average hearing impairment was found to be of the order of 75 db. in the better ear, he had not been provided with a hearing aid and he was some four years retarded in attainment in Reading and Arithmetic. At age 11·7 he was admitted to a school for partially deaf children.

In consideration of cases such as the one outlined above, which are by no means uncommon, the following points may be noted. In the first place, parental suspicion of deafness should never be disregarded or treated lightly. Secondly, expert opinion should be sought whenever there is the slightest doubt that hearing may be impaired. The principal reasons for late diagnosis are probably the lack of screen testing procedures in infancy and at entry to school, and the failure to seek expert opinion at an early stage. The testing of hearing acuity and the recognition of the symptoms of hearing impairment present many complexities. Simple tests of whispered speech or numbers, or of the response to a few isolated sounds, can be highly misleading. That this is so is underlined by the fact that, even where persons experienced in the field of hearing impairment are concerned, difficult and conflicting cases continue to arise when final diagnosis demands great care, and a very thorough investigation of many different factors, such as speech development, understanding of spoken language, intellectual development, educational attainments and family history.

## Age of Onset of Deafness

It is often difficult to decide the age of onset of deafness, but in 34 cases in the research group reliable information was available. In eight cases onset was at birth, in two cases before the age of 1 year, in thirteen cases before the age of 3 years, six cases before the age of 5 years, and in five cases soon after admission to school. Whilst onset may have been more gradual in many of the cases where age of onset was in doubt, there would seem to be sufficient number of cases of onset before school age to support the view that ascertainment of deafness is not made soon enough. The age of onset of deafness is an important factor and can have considerable bearing on the progress a child with impaired hearing is likely to make. What is known about the aetiology of deafness and the examination of data concerning children referred for suspected hearing impairment, would indicate that onset of significant hearing impairment is before school age in the majority of cases. However, the difference between onset at birth and onset in the years before school may be most significant. Even if a child has only been through the preparatory stage of learning to talk before hearing impairment develops, this may be an advantage in the development of speech. In cases where speech has been fully acquired before the onset of hearing impairment, although the quality of speech may tend to deteriorate, the level of comprehension of spoken language and educational attainment may be greatly enhanced. The case history of a child whose hearing impairment developed after the age of 5 years and whose education was continued in an ordinary school, is given below:

CASE C.B. Age 16·0. Private School.

Severe hearing impairment developed after meningitis at age 7 years. He spent a few months at a school for partially deaf children but was then transferred by his parents to a private day school. He does not use a hearing aid as his deafness is too severe to benefit from the amplification provided by an individual aid. His speech is intelligible, but he is a poor lipreader and in communication with him it is often necessary to make use of written instructions and questions. He has received regular weekly tuition at home from a private teacher of the deaf at the expense of the L.E.A. His school progress has been most satisfactory and he has passed in nine subjects at the ordinary level in the General Certificate of Education. He has not tended to make many friends and his handicap discourages participation in many social activities.

This is a case of a child with virtually no residual hearing for speech, but with later onset of deafness, and high native ability, who has made good progress. In all probability his weakness in lipreading may be attributed to the later onset of deafness, as it has

TABLE 6

Average Hearing Impairment in better ear over frequencies 500, 1,000, 2,000, 4,000 c.p.s.

| Average Hearing Impairment (db.) | Number of Pupils | Percentage of Total |
|---|---|---|
| 30–39 | 8 | 11·75 |
| 40–49 | 9 | 13·20 |
| 50–59 | 26 | 38·20 |
| 60–69 | 16 | 23·60 |
| 70–79 | 8 | 11·75 |
| 80–89 | 1 | 1·50 |
| Totals | 68 | 100·00 |

been shown that there is a positive correlation between the length of time that hearing impairment has been present and skill in lipreading (see p. 82).

## Degree of Hearing Impairment

The degree of hearing impairment found in the research group is set out in Table 6. It will be seen that children with impaired hearing attending ordinary schools are not only those with minor defects of hearing, as the average level of hearing impairment for the group is 54 db. In view of what has been said above concerning the age of ascertainment, and the various reasons why these children are attending ordinary schools, this is not an unexpected finding. However, the degree of hearing impairment taken by itself is not of great significance. This is because the figures have been obtained from a calculation of average hearing impairment over the speech frequencies only (see p. 5) and must therefore be examined in relation to the audiogram patterns observed which are detailed in Table 7. The method of taking an average of the hearing impairment in the speech frequencies is only sufficient to give a general guide as it does not take into account the hearing impairment in all frequencies. This is important as, in some cases, impairment in the frequencies above 4,000 c.p.s. may be no greater than for those below, whilst in other cases there may be a much greater impairment for the high frequencies. Moreover, the significance of the degree of hearing impairment can only be fully realised when seen in conjunction with other factors such as speech development and educational achievement. On the other hand a knowledge of the degree of hearing impairment and its pattern, though not the only factor, is essential both for the diagnostician and the educator. In this survey it was rare to find the schools in possession of a copy of the pure tone audiogram made for the child with defective hearing. Whilst it may be true that pure tone audiograms are not easily interpreted by the uninitiated, some indication of the relationship between normal hearing and that of a child with impaired hearing should be available for teachers. Otherwise, if, as happens in some cases, a child has made a good adaptation to his handicap, or has relatively good speech on account of the later onset of deafness, teachers may fail to appreciate the full degree of his hearing impairment. It may also be as well to state here that pure tone audiograms can be unreliable in the sense that, however carefully audiometric testing has been carried out, the results in some cases will be markedly different from previous test results or will be entirely at variance with the child's hearing for speech.

A few such cases were observed in the present study and an example of one is given below:

## CASE S.A.

First referred from his Primary School by a school medical officer at routine inspection at age 10·4. This boy was given a pure tone audiometric test at a Health Centre which showed an average hearing impairment of 45 db. in the better ear. He was referred for further testing at an Audiology Clinic and at age 10·7 was given a second pure tone audiometric test which showed an average hearing impairment of 65 db. in the better ear. At this stage he was referred for further detailed testing at the Department of Audiology and Education of the Deaf, University of Manchester. A third pure tone audiometric test was now given (age 10·9) and this showed an average impairment of 80 db. in the better ear. All of these audiograms were flat in pattern. However, results of speech audiometry were never in agreement with even the least severe of the audiograms obtained. Speech was not defective and he could score almost 100 per cent on monosyllabic word lists at a level of 40 db. without lipreading. Moreover, neither at home nor at school had hearing impairment been suspected. This boy has a twin brother, whose pure tone audiogram showed normal hearing, but even the parents at certain times find it difficult to tell them apart. S.A.'s school attainments, speech and general behaviour were almost identical with those of his twin brother. After a period of over twelve months (at age 11·11) a fourth pure tone audiometric test gave results within normal limits.

Why it is that such variable responses can be obtained in pure tone audiometry is an interesting and important matter that is receiving further investigation. However, it certainly has to be borne in mind when interpreting pure tone audiograms, that results may not always be entirely reliable.

### Type and Pattern of Hearing Impairment

Examination of the type and pattern of hearing impairment in Table 7 shows that 42 of the children in the research group (63 per cent) have high frequency perceptive deafness. Fig. 1 shows a typical audiogram associated with this type of deafness where

FIG. 1.—HIGH FREQUENCY PERCEPTIVE DEAFNESS

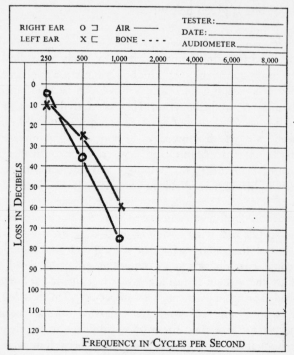

CASE G.J. Girl. Age 11·0. Primary School.

*Cause of Deafness:* Anoxia.

*History:* Age of onset from birth. Suspected by parents at age 18 months. First referred for tests of hearing at age 5 years. Special school recommended but parents unwilling to accept a place. Hearing aid issued but not worn at home or at school.

*Speech:* Serious impairment of speech. Understanding of spoken language: Score 10 per cent on M.J. Lists at 60 db. without lipreading. At 60 db. in classroom with lipreading score 30 per cent.

*Attainments:* Two years retarded in Reading. Fifteen months retarded in Arithmetic.

*Intelligence:* Raven's Matrices (1938) Grade III.★

★ For approximate I.Q. equivalents to Raven's Grades, see Table 14, p. 46.

the response to pure tones is near normal for low frequency sounds, but then drops off very steeply with no response at all to sounds above 1,000 c.p.s. Fig. 2 is of another case of high frequency perceptive deafness where there is poorer hearing for low frequencies but the hearing for high frequencies drops off more

FIG. 2.—HIGH FREQUENCY PERCEPTIVE DEAFNESS

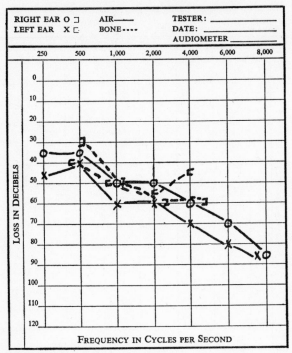

CASE B.C. Boy. Age 9·7. Primary School.

*Cause of Deafness:* Familial.

*History:* Age of onset not certain. First seen for testing of hearing at age 8·8. Hearing aid recommended and help from a peripatetic teacher.

*Speech:* Very noticeably defective in high frequency consonants. Understanding of spoken language: Has great difficulty at 60 db. without lipreading but scores 100 per cent with lipreading at 80 db. (M.J. Word Lists).

*Attainments:* One year ahead in Arithmetic but one year behind in Reading.

*Intelligence:* Raven's Matrices (1938) Grade III.

gradually. A further seventeen children (25 per cent) have perceptive deafness resulting in the so-called flat type of audiogram, an example of which is shown in Fig. 3. In all, 88 per cent of the group have pure perceptive deafness which indicates that, so far as children with impaired hearing in ordinary schools are concerned, we are not only dealing with cases of minor conductive deafness. However it must be stressed that there are many more children in the ordinary schools with slighter conductive hearing

FIG. 3.—FLAT PERCEPTIVE DEAFNESS

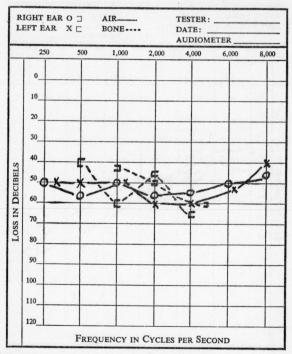

CASE S.P. Girl. Age 12·8. Secondary Modern School.

*Cause of Deafness:* Unknown.

*History:* Deafness suspected by teacher at age 5 years. First seen for testing of hearing and otologic examination at age 12·6. Hearing aid recommended and trial with aid for one year in ordinary school.

*Speech:* Not noticeably defective. Understanding of spoken language: M.J. Word Lists, wearing hearing aid and facing speaker 92 per cent at 60 db.; not wearing aid and facing speaker 68 per cent at 60 db.

*Attainments:* Retarded by about six months in Reading and Arithmetic.

*Intelligence:* Raven's Matrices (1938) Grade II.

impairment than there are with marked perceptive hearing impairment but, as has been noted above, their problems are more of a medical than an educational nature.

The remaining 12 per cent of the group is made up of the less common types of perceptive hearing impairment (where the audiogram is not classifiable as high frequency or flat in pattern), pure conductive or mixed conductive and perceptive hearing

## FIG. 4.—CONDUCTIVE DEAFNESS

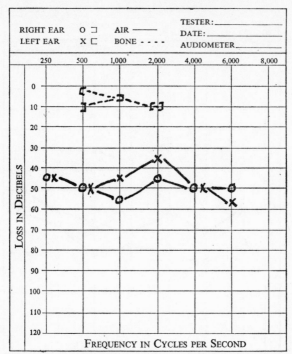

CASE S.R. Girl. Age 5·8. Primary School.

*Cause of Deafness:* Catarrhal otitis media.

*History:* Age of onset uncertain, but deafness noticed soon after entry to school. Referred by County E.N.T. Consultant for investigation of hearing at Manchester University Clinic at age 5·8. No hearing aid issued but medical treatment recommended.

*Speech:* Normal save for slight defect in 's' and 't'.

*Understanding of Spoken Language:* Score 28 per cent on M.J. Lists at 60 db. without lipreading; 76 per cent at 60 db. with lipreading.

*Attainments:* Average attainment in Reading and Arithmetic.

*Intelligence:* Raven's Matrices (1938) Grade III.

impairment. Figs. 4 and 5 show the audiograms in cases of pure conductive and mixed conductive and perceptive hearing impairment observed in this study. Table 7 gives the broad picture of the type and pattern of hearing impairment found amongst the children studied but their audiograms are rarely similar in detail, even within the large number with high frequency perceptive deafness.

FIG. 5.—MIXED CONDUCTIVE AND PERCEPTIVE DEAFNESS

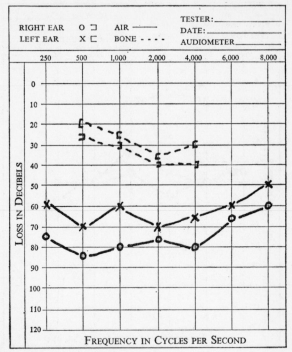

CASE B.S. Girl. Age 10·4. Primary School.

*Cause of Deafness:* Unknown.

*History:* Mother always suspected deafness, tried to teach her child lipreading at age 2·6, but became more certain that deafness was present after entry to school. Tonsillectomy at age 7·0. Seen at Manchester University Clinic at age 9·8 when issue of hearing aid recommended.

*Speech:* Articulation virtually normal.

*Comprehension of Spoken Language:* Score 40 per cent on M.J. Lists at 60 db. with lipreading; 100 per cent at 80 db. with lipreading; 80 per cent at 80 db. without lipreading.

*Attainments:* One year ahead of chronological age in Reading and Arithmetic.

*Intelligence:* Raven's Matrices (1938) Grade III.

There is, unfortunately, little relationship between audiogram patterns and the pathology of hearing impairment. Similarly, owing to the variability of audiogram patterns, it is not practicable to compare the pattern of audiogram with the degree of hearing impairment. How the information in Table 7 is related to other factors, such as speech articulation, understanding of spoken language and educational attainments, will emerge as the further findings are discussed.

TABLE 7

Type and Pattern of Hearing Impairment for 67 Children with Hearing Loss over 30 db.

| Type and Pattern of Hearing Loss | Number of Pupils | Percentage of Total |
|---|---|---|
| Perceptive high frequency | 42 | 63·0 |
| Perceptive flat | 17 | 25·0 |
| Perceptive low | 2 | 3·0 |
| Conductive flat | 2 | 3·0 |
| Conductive low | 1 | 1·5 |
| Mixed flat | 3 | 4·5 |
| Totals | 67* | 100·0 |

\* One case unclassified owing to doubt concerning the reliability of bone conduction responses to pure tones.

*Causes of Deafness*

Table 8 shows the cause of deafness, where known, for all of the group with hearing impairment over 30 db. Table 9 shows the same information for the 42 children in the group with high frequency perceptive deafness. These figures were obtained from examination of case histories and, when these were available, from E.N.T. consultant reports. In many cases discovery of the cause of deafness is often difficult, and exhaustive inquiry fails to elicit any known cause. In this group 22 cases (32·5 per cent) were classified as of unknown causation and this agrees closely with findings in other studies.[1] In 18 cases with a family history of deafness, 13 had siblings with impaired hearing and 5 a history of deafness in other members of the family. These cases have been classified as familial rather than as hereditary, as it was not

[1] Harrison, K., 'Aetiology of Deafness in Childhood', *Modern Educational Treatment of Deafness*, Paper 7.

D

possible to decide whether deafness was present at birth or not. In some of these cases early onset of deafness (i.e. in the infant years) was reported by parents, but not deafness at birth. It is probable that the familial category is made up partly of children with hereditary perceptive deafness and partly of children with familial perceptive deafness of early onset. At any rate it is important to note that such a large number of children in the total group come into this category, for when there is deafness in more than one

TABLE 8

Causes of Deafness for 68 Children with Hearing Impairment of over 30 db.

| Cause of Deafness | Number of Children | Percentage of Total |
|---|---|---|
| Familial | 18 | 26·5 |
| Meningitis | 8 | 11·8 |
| Acute infections | 6 | 8·8 |
| Otitis media | 3 | 4·4 |
| Encephalitis | 1 | 1·5 |
| Anoxia | 1 | 1·5 |
| Rubella | 1 | 1·5 |
| Kernicterus of prematurity | 1 | 1·5 |
| Kernicterus of rhesus incompatability | 1 | 1·5 |
| Causation unknown | 28 | 41·0 |
| Totals | 68 | 100·0 |

Complications of Pregnancy (3) and Premature Births (3) classified as causation unknown.

member of a family, a number of associated factors are often observed. Speech development and comprehension of spoken language is often better than might be expected, in relation to hearing impairment in cases of familial deafness. This may be due to later onset of deafness, or to the help a child receives from parents or siblings. Such children may certainly receive more help in the use of lipreading. It is also probable that there is less chance of maladjustment when deafness is accepted in a family. Special schooling is more likely to be opposed, and may well lead to

## TABLE 9

### Causes of Deafness for 42 Children with High Frequency Perceptive Deafness

| Cause of Deafness | Number of Children | Percentage of Total |
|---|---|---|
| Familial | 16 | 38·0 |
| Meningitis | 5 | 12·0 |
| Acute infections | 5 | 12·0 |
| Anoxia | 1 | 2·4 |
| Rubella | 1 | 2·4 |
| Kernicterus of rhesus incomp. | 1 | 2·4 |
| Kernicterus of Prematurity | 1 | 2·4 |
| Causation unknown | 12 | 28·4 |
| Totals | 42 | 100·0 |

Complications of Pregnancy (2) and Premature Births (2) classified as causation unknown.

maladjustment, if a child is taken from a home where deafness is accepted.

Meningitis was the next largest cause of deafness, but in three cases deafness was considered to be due, not to the disease itself, but to the effect of the drug streptomycin used in its treatment.

Apart from acute infections, the numbers in other aetiological categories were small. Six cases of prematurity or complications at pregnancy were not included in the aetiological categories as it seemed wiser to consider such conditions as concomitant but not necessarily causative factors.

The main interest in these figures lies in the fact that the pattern of causation of deafness amongst children with significant hearing impairment in ordinary schools has changed very considerably in the light of recent knowledge. Moreover where early audiometric testing of children thought to be 'at risk' of deafness is envisaged, some guide is given as to those children who might be included in such a programme.

*Hearing Aids*

At the time school visits were made 46 of the children in the group had been provided with hearing aids. Full details of the use made of hearing aids by these children, and of the various problems connected with the use of hearing aids in ordinary schools will be discussed later. Of the 22 children without hearing aids at the time they were visited in their schools 11 have since been issued with aids and 7 have had the issue of an aid recommended. This leaves only 4 children without hearing aids; 3 of these having an average hearing impairment of 35 db. and one a pure conductive hearing loss. It is clear that virtually all the children in the

TABLE 10

Distribution of Reading Ages for 65 Children with Hearing Impairment over 30 db.

| No. Tested | Ahead of Age | Average | Retarded by | | | | | | |
|---|---|---|---|---|---|---|---|---|---|
| | | | 1 | 2 | 3 | 4 | 5 | 6 | 7 |
| | | | | | | years or more | | | |
| 65 | 9 | 13 | 17 | 11 | 3 | 7 | 3 | 1 | 1 |

TABLE 11

Distribution of Reading Ages and Degree of Hearing Impairment

| Average Hearing Impairment (db.) | Ahead of Age | Average | Retarded by more than | | | | | | | No. Tested |
|---|---|---|---|---|---|---|---|---|---|---|
| | | | 1 | 2 | 3 | 4 | 5 | 6 | 7 | |
| | | | | | | years | | | | |
| 30–39 | 1 | 3 | 3 | 1 | — | — | — | — | — | 8 |
| 40–49 | — | — | 1 | 3 | 1 | 1 | 2 | — | — | 8 |
| 50–59 | 4 | 6 | 5 | 2 | 2 | 3 | 1 | — | 1 | 24 |
| 60–69 | 4 | 2 | 6 | 1 | — | 2 | — | 1 | — | 16 |
| 70 and above | — | 2 | 2 | 4 | — | 1 | — | — | — | 9 |
| | | | | | | | | Total | | 65 |

group come into the category of children considered to require hearing aids. Issue of the Medresco transistor hearing aid to school children only commenced in mid-1958, i.e. a few months before the field work in this study commenced. This accounts for the fact that the issue of hearing aids of a type suitable for and acceptable by school children, was in active progress as the survey proceeded. The first type of hearing aid issued through the National Health Service (the Medresco valve type aid with separate battery container) was too bulky and conspicuous to be generally practicable for school children.

## Educational Attainments

*Reading*. The distribution of reading ages for the group is shown in Table 10. Examination of Table 10 shows that 66 per cent of the group were retarded by from one to seven years in reading ability whilst only 34 per cent were of average or above average ability. 26 per cent have a marked but not serious retardation (between one and two years retarded) and 40 per cent a serious retardation (two years or more retarded). It is immediately obvious that retardation in reading ability (with its subsequent effect on school work in general) is a particular characteristic of children with impaired hearing in ordinary schools. It has been shown in this and other studies[1] that marked backwardness in reading is found very often amongst children in special schools for the deaf and partially deaf and it is evident from the present findings that the same situation exists amongst ordinary school children. Table 11 shows the distribution of reading ages in relation to the degree of hearing impairment amongst the group. This shows that whilst there is retardation in reading for the group as a whole, it does not necessarily follow that the children with the severest hearing impairment are the most backward. There are, for example, 16 children with average hearing impairment between 50 and 69 db. with average or above average ability in reading. Later on further consideration will be given to the characteristics of those children

[1] See Chapter 9. Also *Educational Guidance and the Deaf Child*, Ed. A. W. G. Ewing.

who are succeeding despite their considerable handicap. However, the amount of backwardness in reading found in this study indicates that in any scheme for the treatment of children with impaired hearing some form of remedial teaching is essential.

*Arithmetic.* The distribution of arithmetic ages for the group is shown in Table 12. Examination of Table 12 shows that 56·5 per cent of the group were retarded by from one to six years in arithmetic ability and 43·5 per cent were of average or above average ability. 31·0 per cent show a marked but not serious retardation (between one and two years behind) and 25·5 per cent

TABLE 12

Distribution of Arithmetic Ages for 55 Children with Hearing Impairment over 30 db.

| No. Tested | Ahead of Age | Average | Retarded by more than | | | | | |
|---|---|---|---|---|---|---|---|---|
| | | | 1 | 2 | 3 | 4 | 5 | 6 |
| | | | | | | years | | |
| 55 | 7 | 17 | 17 | 7 | 3 | 1 | 2 | 1 |

TABLE 13

Distribution of Arithmetic Ages and the Degree of Hearing Impairment

| Average Hearing Impairment (db.) | Ahead of Age | Average | Retarded by more than | | | | | | No. Tested |
|---|---|---|---|---|---|---|---|---|---|
| | | | 1 | 2 | 3 | 4 | 5 | 6 | |
| | | | | | | years | | | |
| 30–39 | 2 | 3 | 2 | 1 | — | — | — | — | 8 |
| 40–49 | — | — | 3 | 1 | 2 | — | — | 1 | 7 |
| 50–59 | 2 | 10 | 2 | 4 | 1 | — | 1 | — | 20 |
| 60–69 | 3 | 3 | 5 | 1 | — | — | 1 | — | 13 |
| 70 and above | — | 1 | 5 | — | 1 | — | — | — | 7 |
| | | | | | | | Total | | 55 |

a serious retardation (two years or more behind). These figures show that there is considerable retardation in arithmetic attainment as well as in reading ability. It is true that there are not so many so grossly retarded in arithmetic as in reading, but the number of children with marked retardation is about the same for both subjects. The attainment ages given were obtained from a mechanical arithmetic test, and this form of arithmetic may be thought to be a subject less likely to offer difficulties in itself to the child with impaired hearing. However it is very evident that in fact it does do so, and this is probably due to the failure of the child with impaired hearing to benefit from oral instruction in the subject. In Table 13 the distribution of arithmetic ages in relation to the degree of hearing impairment is shown. Here again, whilst there is retardation in arithmetic for the group as a whole, the children with the severest hearing impairment are not necessarily the most backward. There are 18 children with an average hearing impairment of between 50 and 69 db. with average or above average ability in arithmetic. Nevertheless it is obvious that remedial teaching in arithmetic is necessary for a great many of these children.

## Intelligence

In view of the retardation in reading and arithmetic outlined above, it is necessary to consider the distribution of intelligence amongst the research group. During the course of school visits the Raven's Matrices (1938 Version) was given individually to the majority of the children. This test was used partly because a quick and simple test was required, and partly because a non-verbal test result was considered to be the fairest measure of intelligence for children with impaired hearing. Each of the sixty problems in this test consists of a design or 'Matrix' from which one part has been removed. A testee has to examine the matrix and decide which of the pieces given below the matrix is the right one to complete it. The results of the Progressive Matrices (1938) for the research group are presented in Table 14. From this it will be seen that the distribution of scores for the group is very nearly a normal one. There is thus good reason to suppose that the educational retardation found amongst the children in the research group is more likely to be the result of hearing impairment than of poor intellectual capacity. It is sometimes thought that children

TABLE 14

Results of Progressive Matrices (1938) for 55 Children with Hearing Impairment over 30 db.

|  | Grade I | Grade II | Grade III | Grade IV | Grade V |
|---|---|---|---|---|---|
| Approximate I.Q. Range | 125 & above | 111–124 | 90–100 | 75–89 | below 75 |
| No. of Cases | 6 | 10 | 25 | 10 | 4 |
| Percentage of total | 11·0 | 18·1 | 45·5 | 18·1 | 7·3 |

with impaired hearing are 'dull' rather than deaf. This view is often supported by the speech defect and the quiet, reticent disposition of many such children. Moreover, if their intelligence is assessed by means of group paper and pencil tests, the child with impaired hearing will again make a poor showing. Tests of intelligence that require detailed verbal instructions to be given to a group are by no means suitable for measuring the ability of children with impaired hearing. This is an important point because so many of the group tests of intelligence used in ordinary schools are verbal in nature. Certainly, where hearing impairment is known or suspected it is strongly recommended that a non-verbal or performance scale of intelligence be used as a measure of intellectual capacity.

# CHAPTER IV

# SPEECH DEVELOPMENT AND VERBAL ABILITY

THE nature of the hearing impairment, as measured by pure tone audiometric testing, found amongst the children attending ordinary schools studied in this survey, has been shown in the previous chapter. It has been pointed out that the full significance of the degree and pattern of hearing impairment for any given child may only be fully realised when seen in conjunction with the articulation and fluency of their speech and their ability to understand spoken language. It is standard practice nowadays in audiometric testing to undertake both pure tone audiometry and speech audiometry and, in some audiology clinics, to draw up speech audiograms as well as pure tone audiograms. The reason for this is, that whilst there is a general relationship between hearing for pure tones and facility in articulation of speech, and understanding of spoken language, the relationship may vary according to a number of factors. These will include the age of onset of deafness and the ability of the child to discriminate the various sounds of speech without amplification or visual clues. The ultimate facility in understanding of spoken language will also depend upon skill in lipreading and the amount of benefit derived from a hearing aid. In addition to these factors early training in auditory experience, when given, parental assistance in language development, the level of intelligence of the child and their general environmental experience will have a bearing on linguistic development. There are thus numerous reasons why the pure tone audiogram for any given child is, in itself, only a starting point for a detailed investigation. It is therefore proposed to set against the audiometric data already given, the findings in this study with regard to linguistic development.

## Articulation of Speech

This was assessed on the basis of the following grades. Each child was placed in one of the four grades after discussion between the investigator and their class teacher. In many cases speech was recorded and subsequently studied to facilitate accurate grading.

GRADE A   No noticeable difference in his/her speech from that of other children.

GRADE B   Has slight but noticeable impairment of consonants, e.g. substitutions, omissions or distortions but not so as to make speech indistinct.

GRADE C   Very noticeably a child with defects of speech but intelligible to those familiar with his/her speech.

GRADE D   Speech seriously defective; difficult to understand what he/she is saying.

TABLE 15

Distribution of Articulation Grades

| Grade | A Normal Articulation of Speech | B Noticeable Impairment of Speech | C Marked Impairment of Speech | D Serious Impairment of Speech |
|---|---|---|---|---|
| Number of Pupils | 12 | 26 | 20 | 8 |

TABLE 16

Relationship between Articulation Grades and Type of Hearing Impairment

*Number of Pupils in Articulation Grades*

| Type of Hearing Impairment | A | B | C | D |
|---|---|---|---|---|
| Frequency— | | | | |
| Perceptive High | — | 21 | 15 | 6 |
| Perceptive Flat | 7 | 4 | 2 | 2 |
| Perceptive Low | — | — | 2 | — |
| Conductive Flat | 1 | 1 | — | — |
| Conductive Low | 1 | — | — | — |
| Mixed Flat | 3 | — | 1 | — |

### TABLE 17

Relationship between Articulation Grades and Degree of
Hearing Impairment

*Number of Pupils in Articulation Grades*

| Average Hearing Impairment (db.) | A | B | C | D |
|---|---|---|---|---|
| 30–39 | 2 | 4 | 2 | — |
| 40–49 | 2 | 4 | 2 | — |
| 50–59 | 5 | 15 | 6 | 1 |
| 60–69 | 3 | 3 | 6 | 3 |
| 70–79 | — | — | 4 | 3 |
| 80–89 | — | — | — | 1 |

Table 15 shows the distribution of articulation grades for the children with hearing impairment over 30 db. Tables 16 and 17 show the relationship between the gradings and degree and type of hearing impairment.

These tables confirm two points of interest with regard to the relationship between hearing impairment and speech defect; that the majority of children with hearing impairment over 30 db. will have some noticeable defect of speech but also that a certain number (21·5 per cent in this survey) will have speech that is not noticeably defective in articulation despite marked hearing impairment. Tables 16 and 17 show that where articulation of speech is normal, hearing impairment is more often of the conductive, mixed or perceptive flat type. It is very unlikely that a child with high frequency perceptive hearing impairment will have normal articulation. It is possible to assume that in the case of children with articulation of speech rated as not noticeably different from that of other children, onset of deafness has been after the age at which speech is naturally acquired. Whether this is so it is not possible to say because in six of the cases age of onset of deafness was not known; in the remaining cases age of onset was thought to be at 6 years, 5 years, $4\frac{1}{2}$ years, 3 years (in two cases) and 2 years. Nothing conclusive may be stated from such scanty

information. Moreover there were 10 children with noticeably
defective speech where the age of onset of deafness was thought
to be after the age of 3 years. So far as this study is concerned it
would seem probable that the type and pattern of deafness is
more closely related to normal articulation than age of onset of
deafness.

In consideration of the 54 children with defective articulation,
the majority were not so affected as to make their speech unintelligible and, indeed, those in Grade B were often judged by their
teachers to have normal speech, their speech defect only being
apparent to the listener with experience of defective speech due to
hearing impairment. In other cases in Grade B and in Grades C
and D, speech was recognised as defective but often this was not
thought to be connected with hearing impairment but to be due
rather to malformation of the palate or habitually 'poor' or 'lazy'
speech. It is quite certain that one has to listen to a number of
children with defective speech caused by impaired hearing before
being able to recognise its distinctive nature and most teachers
have experience of only one child with impaired hearing. Whilst
it is obviously important that the type of articulation defect resulting from impaired hearing should be recognised by teachers in
ordinary schools, it is not easily described on paper. It is possible
that this could best be done by means of tape recordings if these
could be made available in training colleges and at special courses
for serving teachers. The child with high frequency impairment
will show defects of articulation particularly in the sounds s, z, sh,
sch, th, ch, p, b, t, d, f, v and h. On the basis of their characteristic
frequencies these are the so-called high frequency sounds and a
child with a significant hearing impairment at 2,000 c.p.s. or
above will have difficulty in discrimination amongst these sounds
and subsequent difficulty in developing these sounds in his own
speech. Thus, to give some rough approximations, such a child
will probably say 'sick' for six, 'ace' for eight and 'stool' for
school. Also he will omit middle and final consonants such as s, t,
d, p and b. The general effect is best described as speech which is
indistinct, in the sense that it lacks clarity, and sounds as if the
child has some obstruction in the mouth or is unable to make full

use of lips, tongue and teeth in the formation of words. When the pattern of the audiogram is flat these errors will be less noticeable or may not occur at all.

It must be remembered that the articulation gradings were based on speech at one particular stage of development for any given child. Improvement in articulation of speech with increasing age, and without special help, was invariably reported by teachers. If all these gradings had been made at age of entry to school in the case of each child the picture would have been quite different. The child with defective hearing at infant school age was often described by teachers as almost unintelligible and sometimes as making noises more like an animal than a child. It is understandable that dullness is often suspected in these children, especially at the age of entry to school.

At the time this survey was carried out no specialist teacher of the deaf was available in the county to give remedial speech training but in many cases children were referred by school medical officers for treatment by the county speech therapists.

Apart from the children graded as D for articulation of speech, all of whom had average hearing impairment over 50 db., the defects amongst the group were in articulation of speech rather than in fluency and sentence structure. The majority of the group had virtually normal facility in spoken language, so far as sentence structure and vocabulary were concerned, and, as has been pointed out, many were rated as normal by their teachers in articulation of speech even though they did, in fact, have slight defects.

The findings of this study tend to show that the ordinary school environment, and the opportunity it offers to the handicapped child for mixing with normally hearing children, lends itself to considerably greater fluency of speech than a special school environment. This was also the finding in the comparative study made by Brereton but it would need further substantiation from larger comparative studies of matched groups of children from ordinary and special schools.[1] It is recommended that a comparative study of this nature should, if at all possible, be

[1] Brereton, B. Le Gay, *The Schooling of Children with Impaired Hearing.*

carried out, in order to indicate more clearly differences in speech development between children with impaired hearing in ordinary schools and special schools.

## Comprehension of Spoken Language

Besides the ability to make himself understood, it is important to know the extent to which the child with impaired hearing can understand spoken language. In speech audiometry, speech itself is used as the testing stimulus, rather than sounds of various frequencies as in pure tone audiometric testing. As a result it is possible to obtain a measure of the child's hearing efficiency for speech. Upon this will depend, in the last resort, his educational and social progress. The measurement of comprehension for speech is, however, a much more complex procedure than the measurement of speech articulation, because the ability to comprehend speech will vary according to a variety of conditions under which speech may be heard. It is necessary to consider hearing for speech with and without the assistance of amplification of speech, lipreading and contextual or situational cues. One has therefore to control the material used for testing, the level of sound intensity at which speech tests are given and the amount of extraneous noise during testing.

In this study two principal measures of the comprehension of spoken language were obtained; the grading of each child into one of a series of comprehension grades for speech heard in the school environment, and a more objective measure of auditory discrimination for speech, obtained under controlled conditions.

The comprehension grades used were as follows:

GRADE A    Readily understands conversational speech without the use of a hearing aid; always understands teacher in class, irrespective of seating position and hears what is said at the school assembly.

GRADE B    As above with the use of a hearing aid or, if without a hearing aid, hears when seating position in class is favourable.

GRADE C  Remarks in conversational speech often have to be repeated, especially if the child is not facing the speaker. Often fails to hear teacher in class; says 'pardon' a lot or misunderstands; doesn't hear what is said at school assembly.

GRADE D  Has great difficulty in understanding what is said to him; rarely comprehends conversational speech and understands little of teacher's instruction in class.

The grades were designed to enable teachers to estimate the facility of each child in understanding spoken language. Table 18 shows the distribution of comprehension grades. Tables 19 and 20 show the relationship between these gradings and the degree and type of hearing impairment. Examination of Table 19 shows that, as with articulation of speech, the perceptive flat, conductive or mixed conductive and perceptive types of deafness are more favourable for the comprehension of spoken language. Only 5 of the 18 children given Grade A for the comprehension of spoken language have high frequency perceptive deafness, as against 37 of the total group with this type of deafness. Table 20 shows that of the 18 children given Grade A for comprehension of spoken language, 12 have average hearing impairment between 50 and 59 db. It must be stressed that these gradings refer to comprehension of spoken language when making use of lipreading and contextual cues and not to hearing for speech alone. Table 21 shows that, when the opportunity to lipread is taken away, the mean score for speech tests of hearing drops off steeply. However, the fact that 36 of the children in the research group have normal, or near normal, facility in the understanding of spoken language with the use either of lipreading or hearing aids, or both, is of considerable importance. It indicates that hearing impairment, even of quite marked degree, is far from being a complete bar to the understanding of speech under ordinary school conditions.

Auditory discrimination for speech was measured by the investigator in the following manner. In order to offset the advantage gained from contextual and situational cues, phonetically balanced lists of words were used for speech audiometry. The

TABLE 18

Distribution of Comprehension Grades

| Grade | A Normal Comprehension of Spoken Language | B Noticeable Impairment of Comprehension | C Marked Impairment of Comprehension | D Serious Impairment of Comprehension |
|---|---|---|---|---|
| Number of pupils | 18 | 18 | 21 | 8 |

TABLE 19

Relationship between Comprehension Grades and Type of Hearing Impairment

*Number of Pupils in Comprehension Grades*

| Type of Hearing Impairment | A | B | C | D |
|---|---|---|---|---|
| Frequency— | | | | |
| Perceptive high | 5 | 17 | 15 | 5 |
| Perceptive flat | 9 | 1 | 3 | 2 |
| Perceptive low | — | — | 1 | 1 |
| Conductive flat | 1 | — | 1 | — |
| Conductive low | 1 | — | — | — |
| Mixed flat | 2 | — | 1 | — |

TABLE 20

Relationship between Comprehension Grades and Degree of Hearing Impairment

*Number of Pupils in Comprehension Grades*

| Average Hearing Impairment (db.) | A | B | C | D |
|---|---|---|---|---|
| 30–39 | 4 | 4 | — | — |
| 40–49 | 1 | 3 | 4 | — |
| 50–59 | 12 | 5 | 6 | 2 |
| 60–69 | 1 | 6 | 5 | 4 |
| 70–79 | — | — | 6 | 1 |
| 80–89 | — | — | 1 | 1 |

M.J. Word Lists used in this study consists of eight lists each made up of twenty-five monosyllabic words.[1] The level of sound intensity at which the words were spoken was controlled by the use of a sound level indicator. The word lists were given by the investigator under three main conditions: unaided and without lipreading, unaided and with lipreading and with the help of a hearing aid and lipreading. In all cases the tests were given either in a quiet room in the school or under actual classroom conditions. When giving speech tests in a quiet room in the schools the distance between the tester and testee was three feet. Under classroom conditions it was not possible to control the distance between tester and testee. It is clear that there are many variables to consider in the giving of speech tests of hearing and, in view of the obvious acoustic and environmental differences found in the schools visited, it is not claimed that the results obtained in this study were obtained under the ideal conditions of a rigorous experimental procedure. However, it is possible to give some indication of the hearing for speech of these children under conditions less artificial than those usually obtaining in the clinical situation.

Table 21 shows the results in speech audiometry for the 46 children with hearing aids at the time school visits were made. Tests were given at several intensity levels but Table 21 shows results for tests given at 60 db. at the ear which is considered to be a reasonable approximation to the sound level of conversational speech. The mean percentage scores are given under each of three conditions.

TABLE 21

Results of Speech Audiometry

| Conditions under which Speech Tests were given | Mean Percentage Score |
| --- | --- |
| No hearing aid and without lipreading | 27·3 |
| No hearing aid but with lipreading | 63·6 |
| With hearing aid and with lipreading | 81·9 |

[1] For details of the design and standardisation of the M.J. Lists, see Watson, T. J., Chapter 12, *Educational Guidance and the Deaf Child*.

E

Table 21 shows how dependent children with impaired hearing are upon lipreading and amplification of speech by means of a hearing aid. The extent to which the children in the group made use of lipreading is of considerable importance. None of the group had been given specific training in lipreading, although those having parents or siblings with impaired hearing would probably have had help from their families. It is clear that children with impaired hearing can become very efficient at lipreading without formal training. Some children who develop special facility in lipreading are able to comprehend spoken language very capably without the need for amplification of speech by means of a hearing aid. Nevertheless, as Table 21 shows, the ideal conditions for the comprehension of spoken language are found when listening through a hearing aid and watching the speaker's face are combined. But Table 21 also shows that lipreading alone leads to a marked improvement in comprehension of spoken language, and children will often wish to depend on lipreading and to dispense with their hearing aids. Efficient lipreading by a child who has not been issued with a hearing aid, or prefers not to wear an aid even when one has been provided, tends to conceal the true degree of his deafness. Teachers are led to believe that such a child cannot have very marked hearing impairment because his ability to comprehend spoken language is so good. For in addition to skill in lipreading, children are also able to make use of contextual and situational cues which further improve their ability to understand spoken language. However, dependence on lipreading and other cues calls for a continuously high level of concentration on conversation and classroom instruction. Moreover there are many situations in school when it is not possible for children to lipread. It is for reasons such as these that, however efficient a lipreader a child may be, he will be that much more efficient at understanding spoken language if he also makes use of a hearing aid.

As with articulation of speech, the comprehension of spoken language is a developing skill, and it has to be remembered that the results in this study are those obtained at one point only in the child's development in this respect. Examination of case histories and discussions with parents and teachers show, that in the pre-school years and the early years in school, language comprehension develops more slowly in the child with impaired hearing. The early years at school are of vital importance for learning in verbal subjects, and even if a child later develops reasonable skill in the comprehension of everyday language, the result of delayed development in the early years may be retardation in Reading, Spelling and written English.

It is important that the effect of hearing impairment on the articulation of speech and the comprehension of spoken language should be fully appreciated by teachers in the ordinary schools. The relationship between the type and degree of hearing impairment and defects in speech development and understanding is not always a straightforward one because of the effect of varying audiogram patterns and the use of lipreading and other cues as an aid to comprehension. There is therefore a need by teachers in the ordinary schools for general guidance in these matters, in order that the effect of hearing impairment on speech development may be recognised and appreciated.

CHAPTER V

# THE USE OF HEARING AIDS

THE use of hearing aids by children attending ordinary schools is
a recent development which has gradually gained impetus since
about 1948 when the first Medresco valve type hearing aids were
made available free under the National Health Scheme. Before
the 1939–45 war some small experiments were made in the use of
individual hearing aids[1] but, as has been pointed out in the introduction to this report, even in 1950 hearing aids were seldom
provided for children in ordinary schools.[2] The first Medresco
hearing aid, with its separate battery container, was, by reason of
its bulk and its conspicuity, not generally acceptable to school
children and the use of individual hearing aids only gained real
impetus when issue to school children of the second Medresco
hearing aid of the smaller transistor type was commenced in
mid-1958. 46 of the children visited in the present survey had been
issued with hearing aids of various types. 34 had only one hearing
aid (13 the Medresco valve type, 19 the Medresco transistor and
2 with commercial aids). 9 had first had a Medresco valve type
aid which was later replaced by a transistor type aid. Three had
both Medresco and commercial type aids. Reasons given for
purchase of commercial hearing aids were either the belief that
they would be more effective than the Medresco type aid or that
they could be worn less conspicuously (e.g. one child used a hearing aid concealed in a hair slide).

The programme of ascertainment of deafness in Cheshire has
been proceeding whilst this survey has been carried out and, at the
time of writing, there are known to be at least 90 children attending ordinary schools in the county who have been issued with
hearing aids. Since in 1957 only 5 children in the county were
reported as having been issued with hearing aids and 12 in years

[1] See the 1938 Report (p. 101 ff.).
[2] *Pupils who are Defective in Hearing.*

58

previous to 1957 the rate of expansion in the use of hearing aids in Cheshire alone has been considerable.[1]

One of the problems which this survey set out to investigate was the value of hearing aids for ordinary school children, and whether hearing aids, once having been issued, were in fact being used and to what extent. The findings show that there are many difficulties yet to be overcome with regard to the efficient use of hearing aids. However, before discussing them, it must be said very clearly that many of the children studied in this survey would not have been able to manage at all in an ordinary school were it not for the regular use of their hearing aids. This will be seen from a number of the illustrative case histories to be given later, and is evident also from the improvement arising in the comprehension of speech when using hearing aids shown in Table 21. In principle the value of hearing aids for children in ordinary schools is indisputable, but their widespread use being in its relatively early stages, it is understandable that problems continue to arise.

*Recommendation for and issue of Hearing Aids*

The procedure at present adopted is that, in the main, hearing aids are issued on the recommendation of E.N.T. or audiological consultants by the Hearing Aid Centres or through Hospital E.N.T. Departments. Hearing Aid Centres were set up under the control of the Regional Hospital Boards for the fitting of hearing aids distributed free under the National Health Scheme. However, there are also many commercial firms which issue hearing aids, either through their own distributing centres in large cities or, in some cases, through independent hearing aid consultants. There are therefore various sources through which hearing aids may be recommended or issued and the main point, so far as the welfare of school children is concerned, is that information concerning the issue of a hearing aid may not necessarily reach the school medical authorities. The nature of hearing aids is such that they do not immediately counteract the effects of deafness as soon as they are fitted, in the same way that spectacles can counteract most visual defects. There is therefore a very great need for training in and

[1] Report of the Principal School Medical Officer for Cheshire, 1957.

supervision of the use of hearing aids by school children after they have been issued. There should be the closest possible liaison between those who recommend and supervise the use of hearing aids and those who issue them. For this reason, whilst the Hearing Aid Centres would seem to be an adequate means for issue of hearing aids to adults, it is doubtful whether this is so in the case of children and issue of hearing aids to school children through commercial firms is even less likely to allow for adequate follow-up procedure. It seems advisable that issue of hearing aids to school children should be made either by the consultant audiology clinics or E.N.T. Departments, or possibly under the direct control of the school medical authorities. In this way better advice concerning the use of hearing aids could be given to parents and children than is able to be given by Hearing Aid Centre technicians, and there would be less likelihood of children being issued with hearing aids without the knowledge of the school medical authorities.

### Use made of Hearing Aids by the Research Group

From Table 22 it can be seen that whereas 57 per cent of children used their hearing aids regularly in school only 17·5 per cent used them regularly at home. It must be noted that at the time these figures were obtained there were no specialist teachers of the deaf employed by the county to supervise the use of hearing aids. It was reported in Hampshire that after supervision by an audiometrician it was found that 50 per cent of the children issued with hearing aids in ordinary schools were making good use of their aids when previously they had hardly been used at all.[1] With the help of the peripatetic teachers of the deaf now available in Cheshire, and with 57 per cent of children already making regular use of hearing aids in school, it should be possible to achieve regular use of hearing aids in school in most cases.

The fact that so few children make use of hearing aids at home is probably because the emphasis placed upon the need for a hearing aid by teachers is not maintained by parents. Reasons given for their children not wearing their aids at home include the

[1] *The Health of the School Child,* 1954 & 1955 (page 115).

possibility that the aid may be broken when at play, that it is only necessary for the aid to be worn in school, or that the child prefers not to be seen with a hearing aid by friends and neighbours. In cases where hearing aids were reported as sometimes worn at home this was invariably when watching television or listening to the radio. In many cases it was found that children did not even take their hearing aids home with them at weekends or after school, but instead left them in their desks in the classroom.

TABLE 22

Frequency of use of Hearing Aids at Home and in School
for 46 children

| | Number of Pupils using Hearing Aids | | | |
| --- | --- | --- | --- | --- |
| | At Home | Percentage of Total | In School | Percentage of Total |
| Never | 19 | 41·5 | 10 | 21·0 |
| Rarely | 6 | 13·0 | 5 | 11·0 |
| Sometimes | 13 | 28·0 | 5 | 11·0 |
| Always | 8 | 17·5 | 26 | 57·0 |
| Totals | 46 | 100·0 | 46 | 100·0 |

The principal reasons for not making use of hearing aids in school were as follows:

Desire not to draw attention to deafness.
Dependence on lipreading and other cues only.
Hearing aid not in working order.
Poor acoustic conditions in school.
Lack of parental co-operation.
Lack of knowledge by teachers about the need for use of hearing aids.

The various motives which lead to a desire not to accept deafness, or not to draw attention to it, are discussed in the section on social adjustment, but as a factor militating against the use of hearing aids it is quite the most important. Dependence on lipreading is an understandable reason for not wishing to wear a hearing aid in view of the considerable facility which some children achieve in this respect. It is necessary to demonstrate to such children the additional help which a hearing aid provides when used in conjunction with lipreading. Also, of course, it is considerably less tiring for a child to have amplification of speech rather than to be continuously on the alert for other cues to the understanding of speech.

Defects in hearing aids were found to be mostly the result of failing to ensure an adequate supply of fresh batteries. One child was found to have the same batteries in his hearing aid as at the time of issue two years previously! The hearing aids themselves were seldom faulty, but sometimes the cord leading to the receiver would need attention or a loosely fitting ear mould lead to the whistling noise due to acoustic feedback. The methods of wearing hearing aids varied considerably and, in many cases, parents and teachers need guidance as to the most suitable place on the clothing on which to clip the hearing aid. It is hardly suitable for example to have the aid in a trouser pocket, as was observed in some cases, or under several layers of clothing.

Only two of the ten children never wearing hearing aids in school gave as a reason difficulties arising from noise level in the classroom. In view of the fact that acoustic conditions are admittedly worse in a school building than in the average home, this is of some interest. But that poor acoustic conditions do not seem to be a principal reason for not using hearing aids is supported by the fact that 57 per cent of those children with hearing aids were able to use them in school without complaint.

Parents often tended to support their children's dislike of wearing a hearing aid in school and, where parents themselves had impaired hearing, to decry the use of an aid altogether. Such parents would state that since they had been able to manage without a hearing aid, why could not their child do so also. Another reason given by parents against the use of hearing aids was the fear that their child would become used to the aid and not be able to do without it. There are also parents simply disinterested and without any particular reason for not encouraging use of a hearing aid. In one such case the child, when asked where his hearing aid was, replied: 'It has been on top of the kitchen cupboard for months.'

At each school visit teachers were asked if they themselves had any knowledge about hearing aids. It was extremely rare to find a teacher with such knowledge. In most cases teachers were very willing to learn the basic facts about hearing aids, but there is also a need for teachers to adopt the correct psychological approach to encourage a child to use a hearing aid. It gives little support to the child with a hearing aid when it is referred to by teachers as 'that contraption' or 'that deaf aid thing', to give two examples of comments heard by the investigator. Undoubtedly greater knowledge on the part of teachers about hearing aids and the best conditions for their use would be of value in increasing the full use of hearing aids by the children in their care. It is suggested that such information could be put forward in the following ways:

(1) By instruction in Teachers' Training Colleges.
(2) By lectures or courses for serving teachers.
(3) By means of leaflets setting out the limitations and advantages of hearing aids, which could accompany the case records of children issued with aids.
(4) By means of illustrated posters about hearing aids.
(5) In the course of school visiting by peripatetic teachers of the deaf.

There will undoubtedly be advances in the design and construction of hearing aids which will increase the extent of their use by children in ordinary schools. In the authorities contributing to the survey of incidence of impaired hearing in this study a total of 1,489 children attending ordinary schools were reported as having been issued with hearing aids.[1] This figure, to which may be added a similar number of children issued with hearing aids in areas not covered in this survey, is likely to be considerably increased in the future.

[1] See Table 2, p. 23.

# CHAPTER VI

# EMOTIONAL STABILITY AND SOCIAL ADJUSTMENT

IT has been shown that children with significantly impaired hearing attending ordinary schools are very often retarded in educational attainments, and may be handicapped by defective speech or have difficulty in the comprehension of spoken language. Concern has been expressed as to the possibility of such children also having problems in social adjustment in an ordinary school environment. In order to determine the effect of impaired hearing on emotional stability and social adjustment, a short questionnaire was designed for completion by the investigator, in discussion with teachers, in the case of each child. An assessment of emotional stability was made by the investigator in the course of interviews held with each child at the time of school visiting. Further information as to social adjustment was obtained from home visits and discussions with parents. As personal visits were possible, this method of assessing emotional stability and social adjustment was preferred to the completion of questionnaires or inventories by teachers independently. The information sought by questionnaires, completed in the manner outlined, is set out below:

What type of relationship does the child form with teachers, parents and other adults?
What type of relationship does the child form with other children?
Details of behaviour in the classroom and playground.
Is his general manner that of a normal child of his age?
Is he exceptionally quiet or withdrawn?
Is he aggressive or is there evidence of lying or stealing?
Does he show any obsessional behaviour?
Does he have any habit disorders?
What attitudes do other children show towards him?
What is the attitude of his parents towards his handicap?

What is his level of attention and concentration during oral and written school work?

Is he regular in school attendance?

On the basis of information obtained in this manner each child was classified into one of the following three grades: Normal, Unsettled, Maladjusted. The decision as to classification into one or other of these grades was made after careful consideration of the case history of general behaviour, the impression obtained from behaviour during testing and interview, and the opinions of teachers. Table 23 shows the distribution of 68 children with average hearing impairment over 30 db. for these grades.

Of the total group 53 per cent were assessed as normal, 38 per cent as unsettled and 9 per cent as maladjusted. The children classified as unsettled were most often described by teachers as quiet, shy, timid, dreamy or reticent. These children were so classified mainly because of their quiet or reticent disposition, and not because of behaviour disorders. In only three cases was stealing or aggressive behaviour reported. Those classified as maladjusted were definitely solitary or withdrawn in their behaviour and were described by teachers in such phrases as 'He lives in a world of his own' or 'He appears to live in a vacuum'. Whilst the extent of serious maladjustment amongst these children is small, the number described as quiet, shy or reticent is considerable. One of the interesting aspects of this syndrome of reticent behaviour is its similarity to that often found in children who are intellectually dull. Moreover the articulatory defects of speech common to the child with impaired hearing are also rather suggestive of dullness. It is probably because of this that teachers are often heard to say of the child with impaired hearing, 'We are baffled by him and cannot decide whether he is deaf or dull.'

Stott has estimated, on the basis of surveys of whole junior and secondary modern schools, or classes, randomly selected from unstreamed junior schools in city, small-town and rural areas, that from 70 to 72 per cent of children in a typical junior school class of forty can be expected to register as well adjusted.[1] By comparison, the figures obtained in this survey show a considerably larger

[1] Stott, D. H., *The Social Adjustment of Children.*

number of unsettled children than one would expect to find amongst randomly selected groups of children.

TABLE 23

Social Adjustment of 68 Children with Average Hearing Impairment over 30 db.

|  | Normal | Unsettled | Maladjusted | Total |
|---|---|---|---|---|
| Boys | 22 | 13 | 2 | 37 |
| Girls | 14 | 13 | 4 | 31 |

That the behaviour characteristics leading to poor social adjustment are the result of hearing impairment is shown by the fact that a child's behaviour may frequently be quite different at home, and may improve rapidly with special educational treatment. One child seen in this survey (a girl aged 8 with an average hearing impairment of 65 db.) was, in fact, so timid and difficult to communicate with when seen by an E.N.T. consultant, that she was considered to be suffering from severe emotional withdrawal rather than from deafness. This child when seen at home by the investigator appeared to all intents and purposes to be quite normal in her social adjustment. It is worth noting that the clinical situation does tend to exaggerate the typically shy and withdrawn nature of the child with impaired hearing—especially in the case of younger children. Schools for the partially deaf are, of course, used to receiving the child from a normal school who has failed to adjust and arrives with marked social adjustment problems, but who soon responds to skilled teaching.

It has always been appreciated that neither children nor their parents are anxious to draw attention to the handicap of deafness. Children with hearing impairment are not noticeably different in appearance from normally hearing children, and for this reason they feel that there is no need to advertise their handicap if it can be avoided. In this survey it has been found that the most important reason for not wearing hearing aids is the fact that a hearing aid draws attention to deafness. When asked why they did not wear their hearing aids children often said: 'It makes me look different' or 'I feel different when I am wearing it'. However, in the many cases where children have been wearing hearing aids regularly in school, it is clear that such feelings are not justified so far as the attitude of other children are concerned. In the case of 46 children, questions were asked about the attitude of other children to a child wearing a hearing aid and in only four cases was teasing or ridicule mentioned. Other children very rapidly get used to the child with a hearing aid and, although there is always initial curiosity, they soon find it no more unusual to see a child with a hearing aid than to see a child wearing spectacles. In the early stages of wearing a hearing aid, the process of acceptance is made easier by simple explanation on the part of the teacher about the hearing aid and the need for it to be worn. However, although this may seem a procedure hardly necessary to mention, it was rarely reported as having been carried out. It is the belief of this investigator that fears about the possible attitude of other children to the handicap of deafness are exaggerated in the minds of partially deaf children, and adverse attitudes are not, in fact, very apparent. This is not always true of teachers' attitudes, some of whom reported their belief that deaf children are by nature obstinate or cunning in the sense that they take advantage of their handicap. It was not at all uncommon for teachers to say about a child: 'I do not think he is as deaf as he makes out to be.' This latter view is understandable when one considers how well some children can adapt to their handicap by making use of lipreading and other cues and so mask the true degree of their hearing impairment.

As an example of how successfully a child can adapt to hearing impairment, it is of interest to give some details of Case TR whose audiogram and case history are shown in Fig. 6.

CASE TR. Boy. Age 13. Grammar School.

This boy is an extremely good lipreader and, when lipreading, has no difficulty in comprehension, except in discriminating between similar sounding words such as 'ship' and 'chip' or 'shop' and 'chop'. Provided he is facing the speaker he can follow conversational speech very accurately, and is able to understand his teachers in the classroom as long as they are facing him. Only the Head Master and Chemistry

Fig. 6

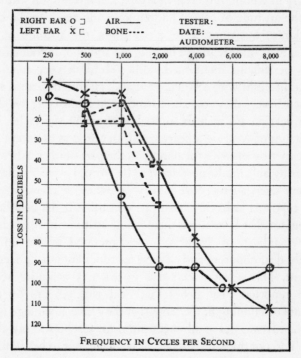

CASE T.R. Boy. Age 12 years, 3 months. Grammar School.

*Cause of Deafness:* Unknown.

*History:* Deafness suspected by parents at age 4 to 5. First seen for testing of hearing and otologic examination at age 8. Seen at County Audiology Clinic at age 12. Recommended to remain in ordinary school with help from a peripatetic teacher of the deaf. No hearing aid recommended.

*Speech:* Noticeably defective in high frequency consonants. Understanding of spoken language near normal when facing speaker; has difficulty when not facing. M.J. Word Lists at 50 db.: facing 92 per cent; not facing 68 per cent.

*Attainments:* In advance of chronological age by 8 months in Reading and 15 months in Arithmetic.

*Intelligence:* Raven's Matrices (1938) Grade II.

Master know that he is deaf, and he said: 'I don't tell anyone that I am deaf unless they ask, and nobody has, not even my best friends.' However he thinks that his friends probably suspect that he is deaf because he has to say 'pardon' a lot when they are talking to him, especially if their voices are low pitched. He claims to hear male voices better than female voices, but prefers a quiet voice to a loud voice. He does have difficulty in hearing announcements at the school assembly, but gets over this problem by asking a friend what has been said when he gets back to the classroom. Though not fond of singing, he joins in singing lessons. He is a sensible and well adjusted child, who makes no complaint about his handicap but accepts it cheerfully. His parents are professional people and adopt the same attitude of acceptance to his deafness that he does. He is of above average intelligence, but it is reported that he only just gained a place at a Grammar School and, in a five-stream school, he is in the E stream.

There are several interesting points about this very typical case of a child with high frequency perceptive deafness who makes a good social adjustment and successfully covers up his disability. He is a bright child with good hearing in the lower frequencies and speech which is not markedly defective. He lipreads well, has a steady temperament, and both he and his parents accept his handicap. However, an important fact is that his educational attainments are not as satisfactory as they might be, and he is only just holding his own in a Grammar School. Moreover this situation may have an adverse effect on his further education.

The factors which have emerged as important for successful adjustment in an ordinary school are the level of intelligence, type of hearing impairment, temperament of the child and parental attitudes. It might be thought that the type of hearing impairment alone in Case T.R. is the most significant factor leading to good social adjustment because hearing impairment in his case is near normal in the lower frequencies, i.e. those most important for understanding speech. Whilst it may be accepted that a hearing impairment which is severe only for the higher frequencies is, as a general rule, likely to be a favourable one for satisfactory adjustment, it is possible for children with more severe hearing impairment over all frequencies to manage well socially in an ordinary school. Case E.A. (Fig. 7) is an example of good social adjustment with a severe hearing impairment over all frequencies. This case shows that degree of hearing impairment, in itself, is not

FIG. 7

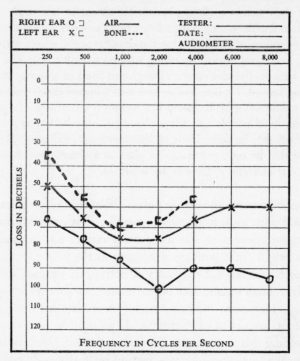

CASE E.A. Girl. Age 10·4. Private School.

*Cause of Deafness:* Maternal rubella.

*History:* Deafness suspected by parents at age 2½. First seen for testing of hearing and otologic examination at 2¾. Issued with hearing aid from age of 3 years and guidance given to parents in its use.

*Speech:* Noticeably defective but easily intelligible. Understanding of spoken language: M.J. Word Lists at 60 db. with lipreading and hearing aid 40 per cent; 80 db. with lipreading and hearing aid 80 per cent.

*Attainments:* Reading: retarded by one year and three months. Arithmetic: retarded by one year and six months.

*Intelligence:* Raven's Matrices (1938) Grade I.

necessarily the key factor in predicting the chance of success in an ordinary school: either in social adjustment, or in educational attainment.

CASE E.A. Girl. Age 10·4. Private School.

A very well adjusted girl of high intelligence with extremely co-operative parents. She had pre-school guidance, and has worn a hearing aid regularly at home since the age of 3 years and subsequently in school. Age of onset of deafness from birth. Her relationships with teachers and other adults are good, and she mixes and plays with other children very well. Her speech, though defective, is easily intelligible and she understands spoken language satisfactorily with the use of her hearing aid and lipreading, at which she is very proficient. She is retarded by one to one and a half years in Reading and Arithmetic.

Important factors in Case E.A. which have led to good social adjustment are, again, high intelligence and parental co-operation. Also, this child and her parents have had guidance from an early age in the management of her handicap. It should be noted that her education has been, throughout, in the smaller classes which are possible in private schools. However, as in Case T.R., even though her social adjustment is good, her educational attainments are not as high as would be expected in the case of an unhandicapped child of her innate ability.

Case P.S. (Fig. 8) is an example of a child failing to make a satisfactory adjustment in an ordinary school.

CASE P.S. Girl. Age 12·2. Secondary Modern School.

This girl is very quiet, timid and frightened. She has a hearing aid, but never wears it either in school or at home. She claims that it makes her feel different, and that she finds it difficult to wear. When the question of wearing her aid is discussed she becomes near to tears. Her mother says: 'She has a "thing" about her aid and prefers not to wear it.' Similarly any mention of special schooling causes both mother and child to be very upset. Special schooling has several times been recommended, but her parents are very anxious that she should not leave home. Her parents have not visited her school to discuss her problems with her teachers. She makes poor relationships with both adults and other children. Educationally she is retarded by over four years in Reading and three years in Arithmetic. Her speech and comprehension of spoken language are seriously affected. On the Raven's Matrices non-verbal test of intelligence she obtains an average score.

The above case history is, in many ways, typical of the child failing to adjust in an ordinary school. Her hearing loss is more pronounced in the speech frequencies, she is of average mental ability, but severely disturbed emotionally. Her parents tend

F

Fig. 8

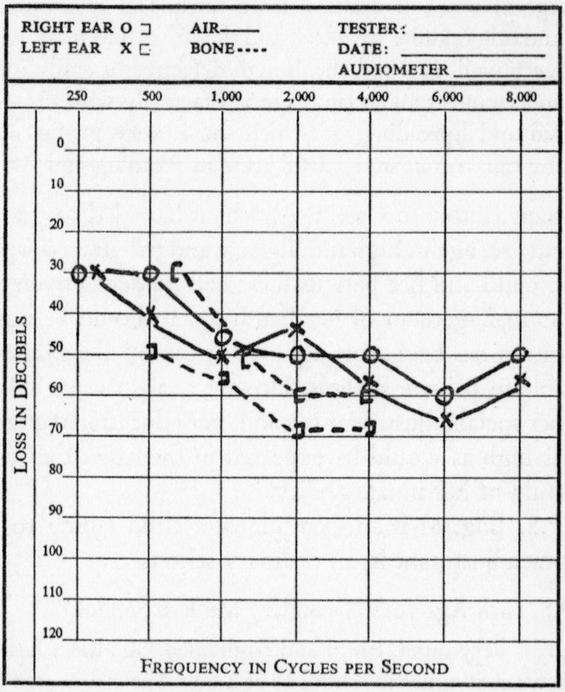

CASE P.S. Girl. Age 12·2. Secondary Modern School.

*Cause of Deafness:* Measles at age 2½ years.

*History:* First referred for testing of hearing and otologic examination at age 8 years. Hearing aid recommended and full-time special education in a school for the partially deaf. Parents would not accept a place in a special school.

*Speech:* Very noticeably defective but intelligible to those familiar with her speech. Understanding of spoken language: M.J. Word Lists 60 db. Unaided with lipreading 40 per cent; unaided without lipreading 20 per cent.

*Attainments:* Retarded in Reading by four years and eight months. Retarded in Arithmetic by one year and eight months.

*Intelligence:* Raven's Matrices (1938) Grade III.

towards over-protection, which magnifies her problems and increases her feelings of anxiety. The result is a child who is seriously retarded educationally, not well settled socially, and, owing to parental opposition to special schooling, likely to leave school poorly fitted for adult life. Alternatively, if her parents eventually decide to accept special schooling, she will be like one

Fig. 9

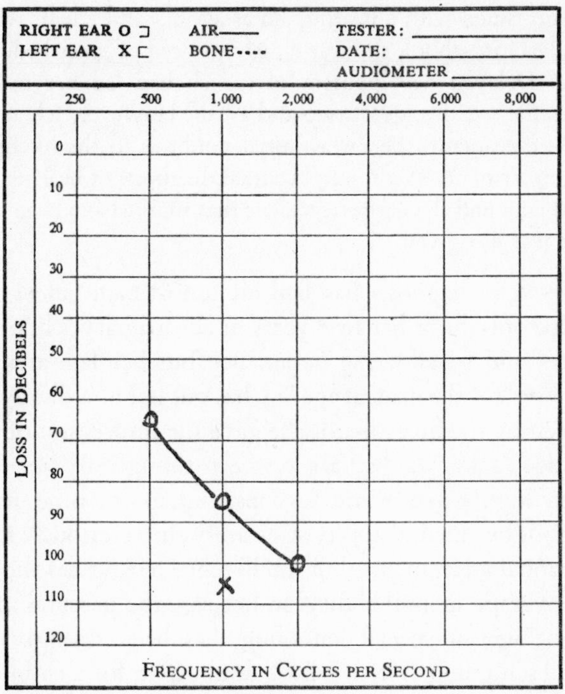

CASE Y.M. Girl. Age 7·4. Primary School.

*Cause of Deafness:* Unknown.

*History:* Mother suspected deafness at age 2½. First referred for tests of hearing at age 5½ but test results inconclusive. Re-tested at age 6 when hearing aid recommended. Seen in her school by present investigator at age 7·4 and special schooling advised.

*Speech:* Very markedly defective; difficult to understand her at all. Understanding of spoken language: With hearing aid and lipreading scores 20 per cent on M.J. Word Lists at 80 db.

*Attainments:* Non-reader. Only able to do mental addition of number. Bottom of a 1st year Junior Class.

*Intelligence:* Raven's Matrices (1938) Grade III.

of many older children who arrive in schools for the partially deaf with marked educational retardation and emotional difficulties.

Case Y.M. (Fig. 9) is another example of a child failing to adjust in an ordinary school and suffering from a severe hearing impairment not diagnosed until a year after entry to school.

CASE Y.M. Girl. Age 7·4. Primary School.

Although issued with a hearing aid at age six and a half, which she used regularly in school, she was clearly in need of special educational treatment. Delayed development of speech had led her mother to suspect deafness at the age of two and a half. However, when seen by an E.N.T. consultant, there was initial doubt as to the likelihood of hearing impairment. As a result, eventual diagnosis of hearing impairment was late, and the early treatment that might have been afforded this child was not given.

Socially late diagnosis has had an unfortunate effect on this child. Not only have her first years in an ordinary school been a depressing and bewildering experience but her late arrival at a special school for the deaf, at age 8·4, has put her at a disadvantage. When seen by the investigator she gave the impression of a timid and puzzled child. She had always been thought by her teachers to be very highly strung and nervous, and, at one time, they had doubt about her mental ability. Certainly she is seriously retarded in educational attainments, but intelligence testing has shown her to be of average mental ability. In her case the parental attitude, whilst not against special schooling, has been strongly against residential schooling. There is little doubt that, for a child already disturbed emotionally by her experiences in an ordinary school, separation from home and parents would not be wise. In her case it has, fortunately, been possible to arrange for daily attendance at a special school for the deaf. One is immediately led to wonder what progress she might have made had her hearing impairment, which in all probability was present from a very early age, been diagnosed earlier. It is very clear that failure to arrange early and suitable school placement of the child with impaired hearing leads not only to educational retardation but also to social maladjustment. It is also the case that the special schools are faced with a more difficult problem when they receive children with severe hearing impairment at late ages. A further disturbing feature of the case under discussion is that, even when Y.M. was finally placed at a special school for the deaf, hardly any of the information concerning her case was made available to the school. There does not always seem to be an arrangement whereby specialists who have seen such children are notified of their admission to special schools.

Therefore vital information concerning the audiological and medical histories of children entering special schools for the deaf and partially deaf is never made known to their teachers. This situation reflects a lack of liaison between those concerned with otological treatment of children with impaired hearing and those dealing with their education. It is suggested that, when a child enters a special school, specialists previously consulted should be notified of this fact, so that they may provide the school with the essential information concerning the child's case history.

Case H.B. (Fig. 10) illustrates some of the effects of parental disregard of medical advice and lack of knowledge on the part of teachers.

CASE H.B. Boy. Age 9·10. Primary School.

The parents of this boy, who has severe high frequency perceptive deafness, showed a general dislike of medical 'interference' in the case of their children (an older son also having impaired hearing) and preferred not to continue with clinical examination. As a result, this child, though known to the school medical authority to have impaired hearing, remained in an ordinary school without any special treatment until he was nearly ten years of age. Onset of deafness was almost certainly before school age. He is retarded educationally, but besides this, his problems are not well understood by his teachers. It was not realised, for example, that his speech defect is related to his hearing impairment. He was reported as being a quiet and withdrawn child, lacking in confidence and showing a 'vacant attitude' towards his school work. Owing to parental objection to special schooling, it has been recommended that a hearing aid should be issued to this boy and that, with help from a peripatetic teacher of the deaf, he should continue for a trial period in an ordinary school.

The risk of social maladjustment arising from hearing impairment is a very real problem. It arises both from the nature of hearing impairment in itself, which is primarily a handicap in language and communication, and from misunderstandings on the part of parents and teachers about the effects of hearing impairment. Much can be done by the staffs of audiology clinics to assist

Fig. 10

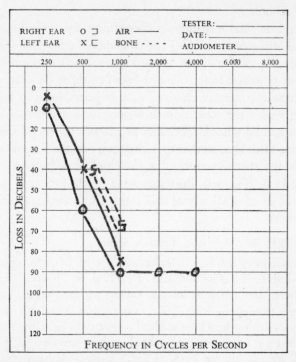

CASE H.B. Boy. Age 9·10. Primary School.

*Cause of Deafness:* Familial.

*History:* Deafness suspected from age of entry to school. First referred for audiometric testing by School Medical Officer at age 7·0 but parents unwilling to
co-operate. Re-tested at an Audiology Clinic at age 9·0 when issue of hearing
aid recommended.

*Speech:* Very noticeably defective in high frequency consonants. Understanding
of spoken language: Unable to score on M.J. Word Lists at 60 db. unaided
without lipreading; unaided but with lipreading scored 36 per cent at 60 db.
and 60 per cent at 70 db.

*Attainments:* Retarded in Reading by two and a half years and in Arithmetic
by one and a half years.

*Intelligence:* Raven's Matrices (1938) Grade III.


parents to accept hearing impairment in their children at the time
the impairment is diagnosed. However a great advantage in
audiology clinics would be the appointment of a social worker
whose especial duty would be directed towards the social adjust-

ment of parents and children faced with the difficulties of hearing impairment.

Peripatetic teachers of the deaf are also in a position to assist parents in this respect, but they have a particular opportunity to help teachers in ordinary schools to understand the difficulties children with impaired hearing may have in making a satisfactory social adjustment.

In the treatment of children with impaired hearing, it is of the first importance that, besides giving consideration to educational progress, attention should also be given to means of ensuring good social adjustment.

# CHAPTER VII

# THE SCHOOLS AND CHILDREN WITH
# IMPAIRED HEARING

In view of the fact that children with impaired hearing are widely scattered in the ordinary schools, it is rare for teachers to have much experience of their characteristics and their needs. Indeed teachers in the ordinary schools cannot be expected to know a great deal about so highly complex and specialised a subject as impaired hearing. Nevertheless some knowledge is necessary if children with impaired hearing are to be recognised by teachers—especially in areas where ascertainment by other means is not thorough. Even when ascertainment procedures ensure that the children are known, the requisite information to deal with their problems must be made known to their teachers who are, after all, the persons in daily contact with them.

To deal first of all with the situation in an area where ascertainment is incomplete; in this case it is necessary for local education authorities to inform the schools in their area of the characteristics of children with impaired hearing so that teachers may be on the lookout for such children.

Tests of hearing should be considered for all children backward in reading and verbal subjects or in their school work generally; their backwardness may be due to causes other than impaired hearing but, as the present study has shown, it is very often a concomitant of impaired hearing.

Children with defective speech should always be considered as possible cases of impaired hearing. Again their speech defect may be due to other causes but, since the recognition of the particular speech defects related to impaired hearing is a skilled task, teachers should ensure that all children with defective speech are tested for hearing.

Where there is a known family history of deafness, or when it is noticed that parents or siblings wear a hearing aid, then the possibility of hearing impairment must be seriously considered.

Children who are known to have difficulty in the discrimination of speech sounds, who are constantly being confused as to verbal instructions or requiring their repetition, should also be suspected of hearing impairment.

Children who are markedly timid and withdrawn, especially if this characteristic is in conjunction with one or more of the above mentioned symptoms, should be referred for tests of hearing. This is because it is very likely that a child who has difficulty in communication due to impaired hearing will be shy, timid and unforthcoming.

The importance of the signs pointing to the possibility of impaired hearing is greater when it is known that the cause cannot be due to intellectual dullness, absence from school or other contributory factors.

It is suggested that information as outlined above be circulated to all schools in a given area so that children suspected of hearing impairment may be referred for special attention, either at a routine medical inspection or at a special clinic.

Where methods of ascertainment of impaired hearing have resulted in a considerable number of handicapped children being known, there is again a need to pass on knowledge about them to the schools. It is of prime importance that the findings of clinical and specialist examination of children with impaired hearing should reach their teachers. It is necessary that the essential findings should be given in writing, but this is only the first step. The need is for persons skilled in dealing with impaired hearing to visit the schools where there are children with impaired hearing and to inform their teachers, at first hand, of their problems. A peripatetic teacher of the deaf is the ideal person to carry out such a task. It is the view of this investigator that school visiting is at least as important a function of the peripatetic teacher as auditory training of children who attend at clinics. At any rate the proportion of their time spent in the schools should be at least equal to the time spent in clinical work. But the efficiency of a system of peripatetic teaching is, of course, greater if the children under the care of each peripatetic teacher is reasonably small. In Cheshire, the provision of two peripatetic teachers is a step forward but more teachers will be required if their services are to be of full value.

Teachers may have very inaccurate ideas as to the nature of impaired hearing. Some suppose that if a child wears a hearing aid he should, therefore, be in a special school. Others feel that the wearing of a hearing aid by a child removes the need for any special treatment. It is misconceptions of this nature that specialist advice can help to remove. Some of the problems of the child with impaired hearing in an ordinary school are discussed below.

Perhaps the attitude of teachers towards the handicapped child is of the first importance. In general it has been found during this study that teachers are invariably most helpful and sympathetic once a child's problems become know to them. If teachers are not fully convinced that a child really has a significant handicap, they will not be prepared to adjust their attitude accordingly. The nature of mpaired hearing is such that its true severity may not always be apparent to the inexperienced observer. Teachers may, for example, be puzzled because a child seems to hear better on some occasions than others. This situation is, of course, to be expected, and is no guide to the degree of deafness. Many factors will allow for variations in the ability of a child to discriminate speech: the noise level in the classroom, the distance between teacher and child, the facility of the child in lipreading, and the general context of verbal instructions. It is therefore essential that teachers should know the degree of handicap present.

It is sometimes supposed that children with impaired hearing are by nature obstinate or that they will, if at all possible, take advantage of their handicap. There is also the belief that children with impaired hearing are less intelligent than normal children. There is no evidence to support these views, but misunderstanding about them can influence the attitude of teachers.

A favourable seating position in the classroom is frequently suggested as a means of assisting the child with impaired hearing. In practice this study has shown that it can often be difficult to arrange for this means of help. In the Junior schools it is generally possible to arrange seating near the front of the class for most lessons. However, in Infant schools, where seating arrangements are less formal, this is not always possible. Even in Junior schools there may sometimes be objections to special seating arrangements if they interfere with the division of the class into sections for some or all of its work. In Secondary schools it may be extremely awkward to arrange favourable seating when children move from classroom to classroom, and are often engaged in lessons of a practical nature which do not call for formal seating. When such difficulties arise it is suggested that, where possible, children should receive individual instructions from their teachers in addition to those given to the class as a group.

It has been shown in the present study that children with impaired hearing in the ordinary schools may often depend to a great extent on lipreading. Lipreading as such is, of course, only one of the means by which children adapt to their handicap. They depend on lipreading plus numerous other cues which they become more or less skilled at interpreting. The facial gestures, tone of voice, and movements of the eyes and body of the speaker, can all give additional clues as to meaning. Some children who are skilful lipreaders may manage remarkably well in an ordinary school for many years, despite a considerable handicap. Teachers may either never be aware of their handicap (as for example in Case T.R.), or may think that such handicap as there is can only be slight.[1] But lipreading is always to a certain extent a matter of chance. Invariably there will be occasions when, because of the position of the teacher, lipreading cannot be used. If the teacher is too far away from the child, as in the school assembly, lipreading is of little value. It is therefore the case that the facts about lipreading need to be known by teachers so that they may ensure that the best opportunities for lipreading are given to the child. Co-operation between teacher and child in the matter of lipreading can add immeasurably to the benefits a child may receive from his own efforts alone. The teacher should always try to make sure that the child is watching him when he speaks, and not to speak until he has the child's attention. The teacher must also be prepared for the child with impaired hearing to position himself so

[1] See p. 68.

that he can see the faces of other children in the class when they are speaking. In the present study cases were observed of children with impaired hearing being corrected for 'unnecessary' turning round in the classroom. In fact, it is often essential for such children to turn and watch the faces of other children as they reply to questions. It is very important that teachers should be aware of the means, other than hearing, by which a child with impaired hearing attempts to understand instructions. For if the significance of lipreading and dependence upon situational and contextual cues is not realised, teachers may underestimate the extent of a child's handicap. It is not uncommon for teachers to make judgments about the degree of a child's hearing loss on the evidence of speech heard on one or two isolated occasions. On such occasions the situation, or the conditions, may have been particularly suitable for the child to make use of hearing and lipreading. Or it may be that teachers will wonder why the child's ability to understand varies from time to time, not appreciating that his ability to understand will vary according to the conditions existing at any given time. It may also be the case that if a child lipreads well, teachers may suppose that he gains little extra help from a hearing aid. It has been pointed out that the concentration required for dependence on lipreading alone is considerable. Therefore, although the advantages of a hearing aid may not be immediately obvious to the teacher the combined effect of lipreading and amplification is very valuable for the child.

Unfortunately not all children with impaired hearing take readily to lipreading. The reasons for this are not clear: research has shown that there is not much correlation between skill in lipreading and intelligence, but that the length of time that a hearing impairment has been present is a factor related to skill in lipreading. However it is plain that a skill of this nature can be improved by training. Teachers should therefore be encouraged to assist the child who does not take easily to lipreading to make use of this aid to understanding. This can be done by improving his capacity for visual observation, and training him to make use of visual clues.

An increasing number of teachers will find that they have in their charge a child who has been issued with a hearing aid. It is never sufficient to give a child a hearing aid without training in its use. A child does not benefit immediately from the use of a hearing aid but requires time to accustom himself to it. Children should have such training at an audiology clinic, or from a peripatetic teacher of the deaf. This is not always possible but, even when training has been given, there is much that a teacher can do to help the child with a hearing aid. Acceptance of the hearing aid by the teacher and other children is, of course, the first essential. It is generally not difficult to satisfy other children's curiosity about a hearing aid, and once this has been done they will usually get used to it very rapidly. Children will often avoid the wearing of a hearing aid, but it requires care on the part of teachers not to force a child to wear a hearing aid. They should try to determine the reasons for the dislike of the aid, and assist the child in overcoming his dislike. Certainly it can do great harm to make an issue about the wearing of a hearing aid in such a way as to draw undue attention to the child in front of other children. It has to be remembered that, particularly in the early stages, a child may be markedly sensitive about the wearing of a hearing aid. Whenever possible a teacher should obtain, from a peripatetic teacher of the deaf, or a hearing aid clinic, some information about the simple faults that may occur in a hearing aid and the remedies he may apply. It is clear that the more a teacher knows about the best conditions for the use of a hearing aid, the more likely the child is to be able to obtain the maximum benefit from it.

Acoustic conditions vary widely from school to school and it may well be that a child with a hearing aid will manage better in some schools than in others. In this study visits were made to schools situated within a few yards of busy main roads. At one school a frequently used railway line runs alongside the classrooms. In some of the older village schools, classes may be separated only by a curtain or other thin partition. Whilst it has not been found in the present study that poor acoustic conditions prevent the use of a hearing aid, it is clear that they must detract from their most beneficial use. In schools close to sources of extraneous noise it may be possible to place a child who uses a hearing aid in the quietest part of the school. In extreme cases, it may even be necessary to consider a change of school. The whole question of classroom noise in the ordinary schools is being investigated further, at the present time, in the Department of Audiology and Education of the Deaf at Manchester University.

In connection with the problems likely to be faced by the child with impaired hearing in the ordinary school, it is strongly recommended that there should be co-operation between school and parents. Parental attitudes are not always fully in favour of the use of a hearing aid by their children. In other cases parents may be unable to accept the fact that their child has impaired hearing. There may sometimes be disagreement between parents as to whether or not their child should wear a hearing aid. Many of these difficulties will be dealt with in discussion between parents and specialist advisers, but it is valuable for teachers to be aware of parental attitudes towards the child with impaired hearing.

It is suggested that Training Colleges might play a greater part in preparing teachers to meet children with impaired hearing in ordinary schools. This would seem to be of considerable importance because of the increase in the number of hearing aids being issued to such children. Moreover it is likely that more children with impaired hearing will be educated in ordinary schools as programmes of early ascertainment and diagnosis increase.

# CHAPTER VIII

# SPECIAL PROVISIONS

*Units for the Partially Deaf*

SINCE 1947, when the first unit for partially deaf children attached to an ordinary school was opened by the London County Council, there has been a considerable increase in this form of provision for children with impaired hearing. The latest available figures show that there are now thirty-five such units in England and Wales and others are projected.[1] All except six of these units have been opened since 1955, so that this form of special educational treatment is a very recent one. A unit may consist of from one to four classes, with an average number of eight pupils in each class; the majority of the units now open consist of one or two classes.

It is generally accepted that units for the partially deaf are in an experimental stage, and there continues to be a considerable amount of discussion amongst teachers of the deaf as to the advantages and disadvantages of this method of helping children with impaired hearing. A detailed report of the units in Reading has been provided by Ling, and other articles have been written by those concerned with the work there.[2] Recently a group of teachers of the deaf working in units for the partially deaf set out their principles and recommendations.[3]

The opportunity was taken by the present investigator to visit a number of units in England and Wales in order to form an independent opinion of their possibilities, and to compare the children in the units visited with those observed in ordinary schools in Cheshire. Details of children attending units for the

[1] List of Schools, Units, etc., for the Deaf and for the Partially Deaf, Nat. Coll. of Teachers of Deaf, 1960.

[2] Ling, D., 'Provision of Services for Deaf Children in Reading', *Teacher of the Deaf*, Vol. 58, No. 343; Annual Reports of the School Med. Officer, Reading, 1955-8.

[3] Memorandum by The Society of Teachers of the Deaf, *Teacher of the Deaf*, Vol. 58, No. 345.

partially deaf were obtained in the course of these personal visits, and discussions were held with the specialist class teachers and head teachers of the schools.

When considering the plan of attaching a small class of children with impaired hearing to an ordinary school, it would appear at once that the children in the unit should be of the same age range as the children in the school to which it is attached. This is generally the case so far as present units are concerned, but one unit visited consists of children of secondary school age attached to a primary school. The Head teacher of the primary school referred to the unit as a 'Downright nuisance' and in view of the many problems which a group of older children in a primary school must produce, this is understandable. One of the basic notions of the unit method of provision is that it should provide an opportunity for the integration of handicapped and unhandicapped children. If the children in the unit and the school to which it is attached are of widely differing ages, integration is hardly to be expected. Provision of units covers the whole age range from the nursery to senior stage, but although most units now open cater for nursery, infant or junior age groups, there are some senior and all-age units. Although local conditions may be against it, the ideal unit both educationally and socially would seem to be one containing children of a single age range only, attached to a school with the same age range. Certainly this would apply to the one class unit where, for various reasons, a wide age range is not desirable; in the case of larger units where the age range would necessarily be wider, the choice of a parent school presents quite a problem from the point of view of age range alone.

A most important point with regard to the setting up of a unit is that the Head teacher of the school to which it is to be attached should be sympathetically inclined towards the principle of integration. Moreover he should be willing to learn something about the nature of hearing impairment, so that he may take an active part in the administration of the unit. This would, at any rate, seem to be necessary if the unit is to be thought of as a class in a school which is as much under the general control of the Head teacher as any other class in the school. It is evident from the findings of the investigator that, in some cases, reasons other than the interest shown in the venture by the Head teacher of the main school have led to the opening of units: for example, the availability of accommodation in a particular school, or its convenience from the point of view of its geographical position. Thus some Heads of schools to which units are attached are not over enthusiastic about them, whilst, in other cases, they have no real control over the unit at all. Indeed, in one unit visited even such minor details as registration and collection of dinner money come under the control of the Head teacher of a nearby special school for deaf children. Since the unhandicapped children with whom integration is desired are under the control of the main school Head teacher, and given that the principle of integration is to be the motive force for the unit, then his overall control of the unit would seem to be essential. If a Head teacher able to undertake the general control of a unit in co-operation with a specialist teacher of the deaf is not available, then a unit may be 'housed' in an ordinary school, but it will not be a part of an ordinary school. On the other hand, it may be argued that control of a unit is best given to the Head teacher of a special school for the deaf or partially deaf within the area, in view of his much wider specialist knowledge of the education of children with impaired hearing. But such a unit is more accurately described as an annexe to a school for the deaf or partially deaf than as a unit attached to an ordinary school. Units at present in existence may be classed as those under the full control of the Head teacher of the main school, those 'housed' in an ordinary school but to all intents and purposes administered by the teacher in charge of the special class, and those under the control of the Head teacher of a special school. Which of these methods of administration is the most satisfactory is a debatable point, but that the unit under the full control of the Head teacher of the main school comes nearest to satisfying the principle of integration is surely beyond dispute.

The three methods of administration referred to above influence the number of children who may be accommodated in a unit. Except for one unit just opened with three pupils, and later to be enlarged, the units visited contained from 8 to 11 pupils in a class.

G

However, as has been pointed out, a unit may consist of several classes attached to one school. If full integration is desired under the control of the Head teacher of the main school, then one class of 8 to 10 pupils would seem the maximum number for a school to accept. Larger numbers, for example 25 children in a three-class unit attached to a school of 300 children, as has been observed, result in too high a ratio of handicapped to unhandicapped children for the average school roll. On the other hand, in a unit of this size it is possible to introduce classification of the children in the unit according to age, ability, hearing impairment and speech development. The single class unit, though ideal in size for purposes of integration, has often been criticised because it may contain children with wide variations in age, ability, hearing impairment and speech development. This situation has been observed and there is little to commend it. In one single class unit visited, there are two children with virtually no speech who would be classified as Grade III under the 1938 Report classification, three with Grade II speech and five with Grade I speech. So far as hearing impairment and speech development are concerned, this one class embraces the whole range of children with impaired hearing from those with the slightest hearing loss to those normally requiring education in a special school for the deaf. The age range in the unit is from 5 to 11 and the spread of ability from I.Q. 52 to I.Q. 98 on the Wechsler Intelligence Scale for Children—two of the class having been classified as E.S.N. by the educational psychologist for the area. This is undeniably an impracticable situation for one teacher of the deaf to be faced with. It is evident that the question of the size of a unit is a complex one, with the advantages of improved classification in the larger units being outweighed by the disadvantage of larger numbers to be integrated in one school.

It was one of the aims of the present investigator to obtain details of the degree of hearing impairment, the intellectual level and the educational attainments of the children observed in units. However, difficulties were met with here, either because audiograms were not available, or records of educational attainments and intelligence were incomplete. In one unit visited, a twenty-two page record form for the purpose of noting these details, contained, in many cases, only the name and date of birth of the child concerned. This lack of information supports the view that whilst a good deal may be achieved in the way of social and speech development in units, this is not always so of educational attainment. If a teacher is not skilled in attainment testing and record keeping, he is not in a position to set about detailed remedial teaching. If he is not fully aware of the degree of their hearing impairment and intellectual development, he has no yardstick by which to estimate what a child could achieve after careful remedial teaching. In another unit visited, there were no reliable intelligence results, and no results of standardised tests of Reading and Arithmetic. However, the teacher of the class estimated that the children were, on average, about two to three years behind in Reading and two years behind in Arithmetic. Since time did not allow for detailed testing by the investigator, it was not possible to obtain sufficient information concerning audiological and educational data to make valid comparisons between children in units for the partially deaf and ordinary schools.

In general, the amount of integration observed between handicapped and unhandicapped children was not remarkable, and was often non-existent. Where integration did take place, it was always partial, and most often for lessons of a practical nature, or for dancing and games. The single child with impaired hearing in an ordinary school may be said to be fully integrated, whereas the child in a unit may often have very little opportunity for mixing with unhandicapped children. The main difficulty is to decide exactly how integration is to be achieved under the circumstances existing. Many of the problems have been pointed out, and are linked with the choice of the main school, the co-operation of the Head teacher, the size of the unit and its age range.

The principle underlying the development of units is that handicapped children should not be separated from unhandicapped children during the vital years of their growth and development, if it can possibly be avoided. This is a sound enough principle, but the problem is how best to achieve this end, and there are those who doubt whether units attached to ordinary schools are the answer. The special school has better opportunities for classification of children into groups according to age and other factors, and has a large staff skilled in a variety of subjects. On the other hand, there are distinct advantages to be gained from the opportunities for mixing with normally hearing children which units for the partially deaf can provide. Especially when the children in the unit, and the school to which it is to be attached, are carefully selected, and full integration is aimed at under a sympathetic Head teacher.

However it is not wise to look upon this matter as one of units versus special schools. It is suggested that there is a place for units, not necessarily as an alternative to special schools, but to cater for:

## 1. *Children of Nursery or Infant School age*

Units attached to ordinary schools for children of nursery and infant school age could play a useful part as diagnostic/educational centres for children ascertained as deaf in pre-school years. A pressing need in the field of hearing impairment is for earlier ascertainment, and an earlier start of education suited to the needs of the individual child. It is one of the difficulties of the schools for the partially deaf that they have a mean age of entry which is on the high side (see Chapter IX, p. 97) and entries often include children of 12 or 13 years with educational retardation and social problems. The bulk of these children come from the ordinary schools. Entry to schools for the partially deaf will be after the age of 5 years, in some cases, because of problems of ascertainment, later onset of deafness and the difficulties of deciding the best placement for younger children whose possible development is uncertain. However, much could be done to ensure earlier and more suitable placement of children with impaired hearing, if units attached to ordinary schools were available for younger children. Units attached to ordinary schools as diagnostic/educational centres for younger children could be a meeting ground for the otologist, audiologist, psychologist and the teacher of the deaf, who could together make decisions as to the most satisfactory placement for children with impaired hearing.

## 2. *Children of Junior School age* (7 *to* 11)

The basis on which children would be placed in units for children of junior school age would depend on their individual needs and would not be made solely on the grounds of hearing impairment. It is suggested that unit placement for children of this age should be thought of as a short-term arrangement, i.e. for children who could eventually return to the ordinary schools. These would be children who, by reason of their hearing impairment, educational attainments and linguistic and social development, need a period of more specialised help than can be given in an ordinary school. Under this scheme, units for children of secondary school age would not be envisaged as, in cases where longer and more intensive educational treatment is required, special schooling would be essential.

## *Peripatetic Teachers*

Another form of provision which has been introduced since the last war and is rapidly increasing, is the employment of peripatetic teachers of the deaf. The latest available figures show that about thirty of these teachers are at present employed by local authorities.[1] The title 'peripatetic teacher of the deaf' is neither very accurate nor very suitable.

It is rather alarming for the parents of a child with impaired hearing who is by no means deaf, to be asked to see a teacher of the deaf. But, whilst they will certainly understand the meaning of the word 'deaf' most parents, and many teachers, are puzzled by the word 'peripatetic'. Whether or not the title could be changed at this stage is uncertain, but some suggestions for a simpler and more positive title are given below:

Teacher of children with Impaired Hearing.
Teacher of Hearing.
Hearing Adviser, Therapist or Counsellor.

The exact nature of the duties for which peripatetic teachers

[1] List of Schools, Units, etc., for the Deaf and for the Partially Deaf.

could best be employed is not finally settled, and local authorities approach the problem in various ways. A major difference is that in some cases the peripatetic teacher is employed by the Health Authorities, and in other cases by the Education Authorities. Since the problems of children with impaired hearing are, of necessity, both medical and educational, this may at once present difficulties, unless there is close liaison between medical and educational staff. An examination of some recent advertisements for peripatetic teachers show that a wide range of duties may be required including:

Assistance with ascertainment of deafness.
Auditory training of pre-school children.
Parent guidance and home visiting.
Formation of special classes.
Specialisation in auditory training.
Division of duties between a special class and with children in ordinary schools.
Follow-up and supervision of children in ordinary schools and advice with regard to the use of hearing aids.

Peripatetic teachers may be asked to work either in audiology units, part-time clinics, special classes, ordinary schools, or in special schools in the follow-up of children admitted to special schools after early training. In many cases several of the above duties would be combined. Generally the age range of the children likely to be seen by the peripatetic teacher would be very wide— from pre-school age to school-leaving age. There would thus seem to be a need to decide whether the duties of a peripatetic teacher should be mainly audiological, mainly educational, or a combination of both. Very recently the appointment of audiologists has been considered by some authorities to deal with such matters as ascertainment, advice as to placement, supervision of the use of hearing aids, and to work in an audiology unit. The word 'audiology' did not come into general use until 1945 and the emergence of audiology as a profession is quite a recent development.[1] The audiologist is usually a non-medical worker whose primary interest is in the measurement of hearing impairment and the rehabilitation of those with impaired hearing. A course leading to a Diploma in Audiology was started in 1958 in the Department of Audiology and the Education of the Deaf, University of Manchester. Where an audiologist is employed it would be possible for a peripatetic teacher to concentrate on remedial teaching and speech improvement, parent guidance and co-operation with and advice to teachers. The findings of the present study have shown that there is considerable educational retardation amongst children with impaired hearing in ordinary schools. The improvement of educational retardation resulting from impaired hearing is a lengthy task, and requires more time than a peripatetic teacher with both audiological and educational duties can provide. The experience of schools for the partially deaf, who receive a large number of children with the degree of educational retardation and social maladjustment found amongst children with impaired hearing in ordinary schools, is that several years of intensive teaching are required to show appreciable improvement. In Cheshire the number of children on the list of each of the two peripatetic teachers is about 60 and, even if they had no duties other than remedial teaching, the time they could devote to each child would be small. Many of these children also require help with lipreading, auditory training and speech improvement. If peripatetic teachers are to be of any real value so far as remedial teaching is concerned, their provision would have to be on a much larger scale. It may well be that the work of the peripatetic teacher should be primarily concerned with auditory training for children of nursery and infant school age and parent guidance. Working in conjunction with an audiologist, they could maintain close liaison with ordinary schools, units for nursery/infant and primary school children and special schools, and assist in decisions as to placement of children with impaired hearing. In the case of children considered suitable for ordinary schooling, their work would be mainly concerned with follow-up procedures, visits to schools and parent and teacher guidance.

[1] Newby, H. A., *Audiology*.

The two principal functions of the peripatetic teacher, under this scheme, would be as an integral part of a system of early ascertainment and careful school placement, and as the specialist teacher supervising those children deemed suitable for ordinary schooling.

# CHAPTER IX

# CHESHIRE COUNTY CHILDREN IN SPECIAL SCHOOLS FOR THE DEAF AND PARTIALLY DEAF

As an extension to the original plan to study a group of children with impaired hearing in ordinary schools, it was decided to make a study of certain Cheshire County children attending special schools for the deaf and partially deaf. Important points had arisen during the course of the work amongst children in ordinary schools, which made it necessary to consider the relative hearing impairment, educational attainment and language development of children in special schools. It was thought particularly desirable to obtain details of such children in order to examine the question of educational placement of children with impaired hearing as a whole. Since there are now several methods of educating children with impaired hearing, i.e. in ordinary schools with hearing aids and help from peripatetic teachers, in units for the partially deaf attached to ordinary schools, and in special schools for the deaf and partially deaf, it is clear that there is more scope for those deciding the best educational placement in any particular case.

There are at present some 120 Cheshire County children attending special schools for the deaf and partially deaf. This represents an incidence of 1 per 1,000 of the total school population of the county, which is the figure already given (Chapter II) as the estimate of those children at present considered to be in need of special schooling. Amongst the twenty L.E.A.'s providing information for the survey of the incidence of impaired hearing, the actual number of children being educated in both types of special school ranged from 0·38 to 1·34 per 1,000 of the total school population. The areas sending smaller numbers to special schools were shown to be either those with units for the partially deaf, or those where the issue of hearing aids to children in ordinary schools had been particularly encouraged. In Cheshire there are at present no units for the partially deaf, and until recently only a small number of children in ordinary schools had been issued with hearing aids. The appointment of two peripatetic teachers of the deaf is also a recent provision. It is probably for these reasons that the number of Cheshire children attending special schools is higher than the mean incidence amongst the twenty local authorities taking part in the present survey (i.e. 0·73 per 1,000).

The majority of Cheshire County children are placed at one of two schools, one for the partially deaf only, and the other for both deaf and partially deaf children. It has for some time been official policy that deaf and partially deaf children should be educated separately, but there are still many special schools educating both grades. The question of grading children with impaired hearing is, of course, a very complex one, and it has been pointed out in this report that, since so many variables have to be considered in placing a child in one or other of the two main grades (i.e. deaf or partially deaf), it is perhaps wiser to talk only of children with impaired hearing, and to dispense with the practice of grading. The findings of the present study reinforce such a standpoint, because it is abundantly clear that grading is not a practical possibility, and the careful consideration of each individual child's requirements is the only alternative.

A number of the children in the two special schools referred to above are over the age of 16 and attend vocational classes. A further group under the age of 5 years were not included in the study. The 76 children here studied were between the ages of 5 years 5 months and 16 years 9 months.

Details of hearing impairment, type and pattern of deafness, aetiology, hearing for and articulation of speech, and attainments in Reading and Arithmetic, were obtained during the course of personal visits to the schools by the present investigator, with the co-operation and assistance of the head and assistant teachers. The findings are set out and discussed below.

## Age of Entry to Special School

The mean age of entry to the special school for the deaf was 5·5 years, and to the school for the partially deaf 8·0 years. The latest age of entry to the school for the deaf was 8·5 years, but there were only two cases of such late entry. At the school for the partially deaf, two children were received at the ages of 10·10 and 10·11 years respectively, one at 11·3 years and one at 12·4 years.

## Aetiology of Deafness

The aetiology of deafness is set out in Table 24, but it will be seen that in 39 cases (51·5 per cent) the cause of deafness is unknown. The largest known categories of aetiology being meningitis (14 cases or 18·4 per cent) and familial deafness (11 cases or 14·4 per cent). In view of the fact that a knowledge of aetiology of deafness is important for the early ascertainment of impaired hearing, it would seem that continued research into the aetiology of deafness is essential.

TABLE 24

Aetiology of Deafness for 76 Children attending Special Schools

| Cause of Deafness | Number of Children | Percentage of Total |
|---|---|---|
| Meningitis | 14 | 18·4 |
| Familial | 11 | 14·4 |
| Maternal rubella | 6 | 7·9 |
| Acute infections | 3 | 3·9 |
| Rhesus incompatibility | 2 | 2·6 |
| Otitis media | 1 | 1·3 |
| Causation unknown | 39 | 51·5 |
| Total | 76 | 100·0 |

## Degree of Hearing Impairment

Table 25 shows the average hearing impairment in the better ear over the frequencies 500, 1,000, 2,000 and 4,000 c.p.s. for the children studied in special schools, set against the figures for the children studied in ordinary schools. On the basis of hearing impairment as measured by hearing for pure tones, it will be seen that there is considerable overlap between the children in ordinary schools and the school for the partially deaf, and between the school for the deaf and the school for the partially deaf. So far as the overlap between partially deaf and deaf children is concerned, this is partly explained by the fact that the school for the deaf has admitted in the past children who, by reason of hearing loss alone, could be graded as partially deaf. The limitations of this system of grading have already been mentioned but, when other factors are taken into account (e.g. hearing for speech, articulation of speech and educational attainments), it is clear that there are still wide variations in the degree of handicap experienced by the children in the school for the deaf. The disadvantage of children with relatively less severe handicaps being educated together with children who are very severely handicapped has often been pointed out before; nevertheless it is extremely important that it should continue to be stressed. More will be said concerning this matter when other data relating to these children has been given.

A further point of interest with regard to the figures in Table 25 is the close similarity between the hearing impairment of the children studied in the ordinary schools, and that of those at present at the school for the partially deaf. The mean hearing impairment for

TABLE 25

Degree of Hearing Impairment for Children in Special Schools

| Mean Hearing Impairment (db.) | Ordinary Schools | School for Partially Deaf | School for Deaf | Both Types of Special School |
|---|---|---|---|---|
| 30– 39 | 8 | 1 | — | 1 |
| 40– 49 | 9 | 8 | 1 | 9 |
| 50– 59 | 26 | 8 | — | 8 |
| 60– 69 | 16 | 5 | 6 | 11 |
| 70– 79 | 7 | 2 | 5 | 7 |
| 80– 89 | 3 | 1 | 8 | 9 |
| 90– 99 | — | 3 | 5 | 8 |
| 100–109 | — | — | 8 | 8 |
| 110–119 | — | — | 8 | 8 |
| No response | — | — | 7 | 7 |
| Totals | 69 | 28 | 48 | 76 |

NOTE: Mean hearing impairment is measured over the frequencies 500, 1,000, 2,000 and 4,000 c.p.s. in the better ear.

the children in ordinary schools is 54 db., and for the children at the school for the partially deaf, 57 db. It is necessary to bear in mind that the figures for the children in ordinary schools refer only to those with average hearing impairment greater than 30 db. in the better ear which, for the purpose of this survey, has been considered the criterion of significant hearing impairment. The essential finding which emerges from a comparison between the hearing impairment of the ordinary school group and the children in the school for the partially deaf, is that there are over twice as many children in the ordinary schools with comparable hearing impairment to the children in the school for the partially deaf. The children studied in ordinary schools were only those known at the time the field work of the survey was carried out, and the ratio of children in the ordinary schools in Cheshire with similar hearing impairment to the children in the school for the partially deaf is, in fact, higher than this. As was shown in Chapter II, the estimated incidence of children with marked bilateral perceptive hearing impairment outside the special schools (i.e. in ordinary schools, other types of special school, or being educated privately) is twice the estimated incidence of children at present considered to require special schooling, both in schools for the deaf and partially deaf: 2 per 1,000 school children as against 1 per 1,000. How this situation arises has been discussed in Chapter III, and some of the reasons for children remaining in ordinary schools have been detailed. The question which arises is whether places in schools for the partially deaf should be increased to cater for all children with hearing impairment comparable to that found in schools for the partially deaf at present, or whether the children in the schools for the partially deaf could be educated in the ordinary schools with special help. Such a question is not easily answered, and has to be considered in the light of other data concerning the relative educational and social progress of children in ordinary schools and special schools.

## Hearing for Speech

It is recognised that, besides a knowledge of a child's hearing for pure tones, as may be shown by the audiogram, it is also necessary to determine hearing for speech. To obtain a measure of hearing for speech, each child studied in the special schools was tested on the M.J. Word Lists (see Chapter IV for a description of this test). Word lists were given under three conditions:

    I Aided hearing with lipreading.
    II Unaided hearing with lipreading.
    III Unaided hearing without lipreading.

The level of intensity at which these speech tests were given was 60 db. (as measured at the ear by means of a sound level indicator), which is a level approximating to that of normal conversational speech. These conditions were chosen as they were similar to those under which the hearing for speech of children in the ordinary schools was tested. It is therefore possible to compare the data for the two groups of children and the mean percentage scores obtained, under the conditions described, are shown below.

TABLE 26

Mean Percentage Scores: M.J. Word Lists

| Condition | I | II | III |
|---|---|---|---|
| Ordinary School Children | 81·9 | 63·6 | 27·3 |
| Special School (Partially Deaf) | 76·3 | 52·9 | 16·4 |
| Special School (Deaf) | 50·9 | 38·7 | 5·6 |

The figures in Table 26 show, as has already been noted (Chapter IV), the improvement in hearing for speech which results from the use of a hearing aid and lipreading together. It is therefore to be regretted that ten of the children tested in the school for the deaf did not have their hearing aids available at the time of testing. It was not possible in these cases to determine the level of facility in hearing for speech which they might have obtained with the use of a hearing aid. As with hearing for pure tones, it is again evident that there is not a great deal of difference in the facility for hearing speech between the children in ordinary schools and the children in the school for the partially deaf. On the other hand, speech tests given at a level of intensity of 60 db. present considerable difficulty to children in the school for the deaf. However there is still an overlap in this respect between the groups, in that six of the children in the school for the deaf showed better hearing for speech than the mean for children in the school for the partially deaf, and two showed better hearing for speech than the mean for children in ordinary schools. Similarly, five of the children in the school for the partially deaf showed better hearing for speech than the mean for children in the ordinary schools.

## Articulation of Speech

Owing to the wide range of hearing impairment amongst the children in the special schools, it was not practicable to measure the articulation of speech by the method adopted for the children in ordinary schools. A special five-point scale was devised and teachers were asked to place each child in one of the following grades:

A Spontaneous speech—talks in sentences that constitute continuous sound patterns, normal intonation and rhythm.

B As for A but with imperfect intonation and rhythm.

C Talks in sentences that consist of separately uttered words rather than continuous patterns.

D Tends to talk in single words which are intelligible to those who know the child.

E Utters very imperfect approximations to normal words— very often unintelligible.

The distribution of the children in special schools for these grades is shown in Table 27. The comparative measurement of articulation of speech is a difficult matter, and the method of grading used here does not permit of any valid comparison between the children in ordinary schools and special schools. Between the school for the deaf and the school for the partially deaf there is again some degree of overlap. However, it is clear that articulation of speech amongst the children in the school for the deaf is considerably more defective than amongst those in the school for the partially deaf. This is understandably so, in view of the presence of a number of very deaf children in the school for the deaf. 15 of the children in the school for the deaf would not, by speech alone, be able to make themselves understood, and a further 19 could only be understood with difficulty. It is partly for this reason that these children often make use of sign language or finger spelling when communicating with each other. On the other hand, there are fourteen children in the school for the deaf whose articulation of speech was rated as equivalent to that of the majority of the children in the school for the partially deaf. Differences of this degree in speech development are a further argument against educating together children with too wide a range of handicap.

TABLE 27

Articulation of Speech for 76 Children attending Special Schools

| Grade | School for Deaf | School for Partially Deaf |
|---|---|---|
| A | 6 | 6 |
| B | 8 | 18 |
| C | 19 | 4 |
| D | 8 | — |
| E | 7 | — |

## Educational Attainments

*Reading.* Each child attending a special school was tested individually using the Schonell Graded Word Reading Test. This test was also used with the children attending ordinary schools. The distribution of reading ages for the children in special schools and ordinary schools is set out below.

*Arithmetic.* To obtain a measure of attainment in this subject each child was tested by means of the Schonell Essential Mechanical Arithmetic Test. This test was also used with the children attending ordinary schools. The distribution of arithmetic ages for the children in special schools and ordinary schools is set out below.

Examination of the attainments in Reading and Arithmetic

## TABLE 28
### Attainment in Reading

| | Number Tested | Ahead of Average | Average | Retarded by more than years | | | | | | | | |
| --- | --- | --- | --- | --- | --- | --- | --- | --- | --- | --- | --- | --- |
| | | | | 1 | 2 | 3 | 4 | 5 | 6 | 7 | 8 | 9 |
| Ordinary School | 65 | 9 | 13 | 17 | 11 | 3 | 7 | 3 | 1 | 1 | — | — |
| School for Partially Deaf | 26 | 1 | 4 | 3 | 7 | 1 | 5 | 3 | 1 | 1 | — | — |
| School for Deaf | 44 | — | 3 | — | 8 | 4 | 7 | 6 | 7 | 7 | 1 | 1 |

### Comparison of Reading Attainments

| | Percentage Average or above | Percentage 1 to 2 years behind | Percentage over 2 years behind |
| --- | --- | --- | --- |
| Ordinary School | 34 | 26 | 40 |
| School for Partially Deaf | 19 | 12 | 69 |
| School for Deaf | 7 | — | 93 |

## TABLE 29
### Attainment in Arithmetic

| | Number Tested | Ahead of Average | Average | Retarded by more than years | | | | | | |
| --- | --- | --- | --- | --- | --- | --- | --- | --- | --- | --- |
| | | | | 1 | 2 | 3 | 4 | 5 | 6 | 7 |
| Ordinary School | 55 | 7 | 17 | 17 | 7 | 3 | 1 | 2 | 1 | — |
| School for Partially Deaf | 23 | 1 | 5 | 6 | 5 | 5 | — | 1 | — | — |
| School for Deaf | 42 | — | 3 | 5 | 7 | 4 | 8 | 11 | 2 | 2 |

### Comparison of Arithmetic Attainment

| | Percentage Average or above | Percentage 1 to 2 years behind | Percentage over 2 years behind |
| --- | --- | --- | --- |
| Ordinary School | 43·5 | 31·0 | 25·5 |
| School for Partially Deaf | 26·0 | 26·0 | 48·0 |
| School for Deaf | 7·0 | 12·0 | 81·0 |

of the special school children shows a serious amount of retardation. From Tables 28 and 29, it will be seen that the percentages of children in the school for the partially deaf retarded by two years or more in Reading and Arithmetic are greater than those for children in the ordinary schools. Similarly there are less children with average or above average attainment in these subjects in the school for the partially deaf than in the ordinary schools. As has been shown in Table 25, there is little difference in hearing impairment between the two groups. This also applies to innate ability, as shown by the following results in the Raven's Matrices Test for the children in the school for the partially deaf:

| Grade | I | II | III | IV | V |
|---|---|---|---|---|---|
| No. of cases | 3 | 6 | 8 | 6 | I |
| Percentage of Total | 12·5 | 25·0 | 33·5 | 25·0 | 4·0 |

Nor is it the case that children with high attainment are returned to ordinary schools, only two Cheshire County children having been returned from the school for the partially deaf to ordinary schools over the last four years. It has to be remembered that the mean age of entry to the school for the partially deaf is 8 years, and it is possible that the children most obviously failing in their school work are the ones most likely to be referred for special schooling, and often at a late age. However, there are various reasons why children remain in ordinary schools, reasons not always related to their progress in school work.[1] If late entry to the special school is a deciding factor in the level of achievement likely to be reached, placement in the school for the partially deaf from the age of 7 and upwards would appear to be of little benefit educationally. Further investigation is necessary to determine the exact reasons for the disparity in educational attainment between children in the school for the partially deaf and children in the ordinary schools. It may reasonably be thought that children educated in small classes by specialist teachers should do at least as well, educationally, as children with comparable hearing impairment in ordinary schools.

[1] See Table 5, p. 28.

Educational attainment is not, of course, the only factor with which special schools are concerned. There is also the question of social adjustment. It has not been possible in this survey to carry out a full comparison of social adjustment amongst children in special schools and ordinary schools. However, in ten cases, children observed in ordinary schools before transfer to the special school, were subsequently observed in the special school for the partially deaf. It was noticeable that the syndrome of timidity and withdrawal found to be common amongst the children with impaired hearing in the ordinary schools (see Chapter VI) was no longer evident amongst these children. It is felt that this is a direct result of the fact that their handicap is understood by the staff of the special school, and that the children therefore feel accepted. Moreover, they are together with children who have similar handicaps, and this is likely to lead to a better understanding amongst the children themselves. Lack of knowledge of the symptoms of hearing impairment and of the difficulties with which the handicapped child is confronted is common amongst teachers in the ordinary schools. This is understandable, for few teachers have the requisite information, but, unwittingly, it can lead to a misunderstanding of the handicapped child, e.g. that he is dull or obstinate or takes advantage of his handicap. If a larger number of children with impaired hearing were, in the future, to be recommended for education in ordinary schools, then particular attention would have to be given to the problem of how best to inform teachers of their difficulties. This would be essential if social maladjustment is to be avoided. The peripatetic teacher system is a possible means of keeping teachers informed about handicapped children in their charge, but an adequate number of such teachers would have to be available. It is likely that, in any case, their work would need to be supplemented by special courses for teachers with a handicapped child in their school, and by the use of instructional posters and leaflets about hearing impairment and the use of hearing aids.

Comparison of the attainments of children in the school for the deaf and the ordinary schools is not, of course, valid for those children with more severe handicaps than are found amongst ordinary school children. However the hearing impairment, educational attainment and intellectual development of the six children in the school for the deaf with the least severe handicap is set out in Table 30. Also shown in Table 30 are similar details for six children with comparable hearing impairment who are attending ordinary schools. Matching of groups of children from ordinary and special schools is a difficult procedure, and, in this survey, time did not allow the bringing together of large groups of children matched for age, hearing impairment and intellectual development. Nevertheless, Table 30 shows that whilst there is evidence that some children in the ordinary schools make satisfactory progress educationally, the same cannot be said for any of the children with comparable hearing impairment observed in this survey in the school for the deaf. It is not claimed that all children with this degree of hearing impairment will do well in the ordinary schools. Table 30 is of most importance because it shows that children who might well have been expected to do better than children in the ordinary schools, in view of the special arrangements made for their education, have not, in fact, done so.

The primary purpose of this part of the survey has been to determine the relative progress of the children in special schools and ordinary schools. A further investigation is required into the reasons for the disparity in attainment of the two groups in Table 30. It is therefore only proposed to deal briefly with some possibilities. Differences in age of onset of deafness between the groups might have been considered an important factor. However, in all the cases of children in ordinary schools, deafness was noticed before entry to school. Also the difference in innate ability between the groups is not marked; though two children in the school for the deaf obtained a below average score on the Raven's Matrices Test. It is possible that the combined effect of segregation from hearing children, and education together with children having very severe hearing impairment is a factor leading to educational retardation. It is also likely that the standards aimed at in the school for the deaf are low, and that this has a depressing effect on the attainments of the children in the school with less

TABLE 30

Comparison of Attainments of Children in Ordinary and
Special School

Ordinary School

| Child | Age | Average Hearing Impairment | I.Q. | R.A. | A.A. | Number of Years at Special School |
|-------|-----|------|------|------|------|------|
| A | 10·3 | 60 | C+ | 12·2 | 9·9 | — |
| B | 13·7 | 60 | C | 12·7 | 12·7 | — |
| C | 11·7 | 60 | B | 9·4 | 14·3 | — |
| D | 12·6 | 60 | C | 14·8 | 15·9 | — |
| E | 10·4 | 60 | C | 10·9 | 10·11 | — |
| F | 9·8 | 65 | C | 10·9 | 10·11 | — |

Special School

| Child | Age | Average Hearing Impairment | I.Q. | R.A. | A.A. | Number of Years at Special School |
|-------|-----|------|------|------|------|------|
| A | 10·0 | 60 | C+ | 7·10 | 8·6 | 4·3 |
| B | 13·10 | 60 | D | 7·2 | 8·1 | 7·0 |
| C | 13·1 | 65 | C | 9·8 | 11·0 | 5·9 |
| D | 13·9 | 65 | C− | 8·3 | 9·6 | 7·0 |
| E | 13·10 | 65 | C− | 8·2 | 8·8 | 8·0 |
| F | 16·0 | 60 | C | 9·7 | 11·4 | 11·4 |

KEY

R.A. Reading Age.        A.A. Arithmetic Age.
I.Q. based on score obtained on Raven's Matrices Test (1938 Version):
    B Above Average; C+ High Average; C Average; C− Low Average;
    D Below Average.

severe handicaps. Further reasons for retardation might be sought
in teaching methods, and in the use made of group and individual
hearing aids.

## Educational Placement

Many factors other than those covered in this Chapter would
have to be considered in discussing the implications of the findings.
The point of view of those faced with the day to day problems
of the education of the deaf cannot adequately be expressed here.
Nor is it necessarily the case that generalizations can be made
from the results of a small survey of this nature. However it is

proposed to make one or two tentative suggestions, based on the trend shown by the present findings.

It would seem a matter of urgency that steps should immediately be taken to hasten the separate education of children with marked difference in the degree of their handicap. More agreement is necessary as to the criterion on which referral for special schooling should be based. Serious consideration should be given to the possibility of providing education in the ordinary schools for certain of the children at present considered to require special schooling in the school for the partially deaf. The increase in the use of hearing aids in ordinary schools, and in the provision of peripatetic teachers of the deaf, and units attached to ordinary schools, might well enable a greater number of children with impaired hearing to benefit from education in the ordinary schools.

# CHAPTER X

# PLANNING EDUCATIONAL PROVISION

THE planning of educational provision for children with impaired hearing has, in recent years, become very much more comprehensive in nature. It is not only those children so severely handicapped as to require special schooling that demand attention. Owing to the considerable range in the degree of deafness from which a child may suffer it is necessary to make provision for many different degrees of handicap. Interest has increased in children with impaired hearing in ordinary schools, both state controlled and independent, in various types of special school, in occupation centres and hospitals, and in pre-school children with impaired hearing. It is therefore necessary for L.E.A.'s to design a comprehensive scheme to cover the needs of all types of children with impaired hearing in their area.

Any scheme to deal with hearing impairment must be based on accurate ascertainment at as early an age as possible. Screening tests of hearing for pre-school children, mostly carried out by specially trained health visitors, form the basis of early ascertainment. However not all forms of deafness are present at birth, or develop during pre-school years, and further screening by the sweep frequency technique is desirable at later ages. Gramophone audiometry is still in use for children of 8 years and over, but is gradually being replaced by the sweep frequency technique, which has been shown to be far superior.[1] From returns provided by L.E.A.'s during the course of the present survey, it is apparent that either 5 years of age or 8 years, or both, is the most common time for school age screening tests. So far as pre-school children are concerned, some authorities consider the testing of whole age groups too ambitious a scheme, and prefer to test only those children who are 'at risk' of deafness from pre-natal or peri-natal causes, or family history, or who are late in developing

[1] *Educational Guidance and the Deaf Child*, Chapter 5.

speech. Routine audiometric testing of age groups does however seem to be essential for school age children. Various studies have shown that teachers only do slightly better than chance in detecting hearing loss.[1] The present study has shown that teachers will often be uncertain as to the presence of hearing impairment amongst their pupils, and may even doubt it when it has been diagnosed if, as often happens, a child adapts well to his handicap. If, however, referral of 'suspects' only is envisaged, and their examination carried out initially at routine school medical inspections, then the following children should be considered: catarrhal children or those with running or discharging ears; those failing to respond to commands at certain times or in certain places; those inexplicably retarded in their school work and especially in reading and verbal subjects; those frequently saying 'pardon' or failing to understand instructions; those unduly quiet, apathetic or withdrawn; those with family history of deafness and (above all) those whose speech is anything but absolutely normal with regard to articulation, especially with regard to the formation of certain consonants such as 's' and 't'. Speech defects of this nature should be particularly watched for at the age of entry to school.

Any thorough programme of ascertainment calls for trained staff and special equipment, and there are still parts of the country where neither are available. Clinics with acoustically treated rooms are required for the further testing and diagnosis of children who fail initial screening tests.[2] The measurement of hearing is a skilled task, and results of pure tone and speech audiometry need careful interpretation. It is therefore recommended that at least one full-time audiologist should be employed by local authorities to undertake hearing tests of children who have failed initial screening tests. Such a worker would also be in a position to advise and assist in the co-ordination of a comprehensive scheme for all children with impaired hearing of pre-school and school age. Examination by an E.N.T. consultant is considered essential for

[1] Curry, E. T., 'Are Teachers Good Judges of Pupils' Hearing?', *Journal of Exceptional Children*, Vol. 21, 1954.

[2] For notes on the design of audiology clinics, see John, J. E. J., 'Audiology Clinics', *Medical Officer*, Vol. 105, No. 3, Jan. 1961.

every child who is shown, by detailed audiometric testing, to have a significant impairment of hearing. A decision may then be taken as to whether medical treatment is possible. Differential diagnosis may be required where emotional disturbance is suspected, or intellectual development is retarded. In such cases it would be necessary for the services of a psychologist to be available.

The lack of an adequate programme of ascertainment means that children with undiagnosed hearing impairment will, inevitably, continue to be found in the ordinary schools. The figures obtained in this study as to ages at first referral for suspected hearing impairment (see p. 29) help to underline this point. In Cheshire, where a comprehensive scheme of ascertainment has been in progress for the past two years, the number of children known to have hearing impairment steadily increases. It is clear that accurate ascertainment must precede any scheme for educational provision or medical treatment. Unless there is early ascertainment, pre-school guidance to parents and children, which has been shown in this study to be of great value for success in school, cannot be provided.

In conjunction with ascertainment programmes it is necessary to have accurate central records of children with impaired hearing. Moreover, liaison between the school medical authorities and the schools is essential if the information obtained by specialist consultants is to reach the teachers. A very clear finding of the present study has been that teachers often have no written information concerning the children who have been seen by various specialists. This is particularly so in the case of the results of hearing tests. It is therefore suggested that the following details be provided for the teacher of a child seen at an audiology clinic:

## RECORD FORM FOR CHILDREN SEEN IN AUDIOLOGY CLINICS

To Head Teacher.......................................School
............ was referred to.............................Clinic
for audiometric testing and the following information is given for your guidance in his/her educational treatment:

HEARING IMPAIRMENT: A summary of results of pure tone testing and

H*

speech audiometry, and notes on any defects of speech resulting from the hearing impairment.

RESULTS of psychological or attainment tests if these have been obtained.

Details of the hearing aid, if one is issued, with information as to the necessity for wearing a hearing aid.

Any points which would be of value to the teacher in education of the child, e.g. suggested position in class, degree of facility the child has in lipreading, need for both listening and watching for the child with a hearing aid.

Information with regard to any guidance which is being given to the parents in making best use of the hearing aid, i.e. at home as well as school.

The investigations carried out amongst ordinary school children in Cheshire have shown that, for various reasons, children with severe hearing impairment may remain in the ordinary schools. Many of the children with significant bilateral perceptive hearing impairment found in ordinary schools in Cheshire are similar in degree of hearing impairment to children in schools for the partially deaf. It cannot be assumed that all the children with impaired hearing in ordinary schools will have a less severe impairment than is found amongst children in special schools. This situation could undoubtedly be improved by earlier ascertainment and diagnosis, but in view of later onset of deafness in certain cases, difficulty in decisions as to placement in borderline cases, and parental refusal to accept special school places, there will always be some children with severe hearing impairment in the ordinary schools. But the child with significant hearing impairment in an ordinary school, whether there by accident or design, cannot manage without some form of special help.

Whatever special help is provided should be commenced as early as possible if educational retardation and social maladjustment is to be avoided. This is particularly so in the case of the provision of hearing aids. It has been shown in this study how great a help a hearing aid may be to the child with impaired hearing in an ordinary school, despite poor acoustic conditions.

The quieter the conditions, the more help a hearing aid may be in the discrimination of speech, but in everyday school conditions it is still possible for a child to obtain invaluable assistance from a hearing aid. However, a hearing aid should be worn from as early an age as possible. It is now well accepted that even very young children can benefit from the use of a hearing aid. The earlier a child becomes used to the idea of wearing a hearing aid the better. There is no reason why the child with impaired hearing should not wear a hearing aid from the age of entry to school. Indeed, where onset of deafness is at birth or in the early years, hearing aids are commonly issued to pre-school children and used with advantage.

But it is clear that children issued with hearing aids do not necessarily use them. This is due partly to inadequate instruction and guidance to parents when hearing aids are issued, and partly to lack of subsequent follow-up procedures to make sure that hearing aids are being used effectively. It has been pointed out that the present method of issue of hearing aids does not guarantee adequate instruction in their use for parents. Moreover, since the issue of a hearing aid does not always become known to the school medical authorities, follow-up procedures cannot be put into effect.

It is therefore recommended that issue of the Medresco hearing aids to school children should be under the control of the Principal School Medical Officer for any given area. Alternatively, no child of school age should be issued with a hearing aid, either through a Hearing Aid Centre or privately, without the appropriate school medical authority being informed.

Psychological factors responsible for failure to use hearing aids constitute a challenge to school medical officers, peripatetic teachers and teachers in ordinary schools, in encouraging their acceptance.

Further advances will continue to be made in the design of individual hearing aids, but the problem of poor acoustics in ordinary schools will remain. As one means of overcoming this problem, it is possible that experiments might be made in the use of hearing aids which can be used in conjunction with an inductance loop system in ordinary school classrooms. This type of provision is common in units for the partially deaf attached to ordinary schools, but it is worth considering whether it could be used even when only one or two children with impaired hearing are enrolled in an ordinary class. It would be necessary for the teacher to use a microphone, but there would be very distinct advantages in that the level of amplification of his speech could be suitably adjusted and held constant. Moreover the child with impaired hearing would not be at a disadvantage, as he frequently is, when the teacher is in such a position as to prevent the use of lipreading. The cost of a simple inductance loop system is not great, and it could be moved into another classroom at the end of each school year if the children using it have to change class-rooms. This system would, of course, be less practicable in second-ary schools where changes of classroom are more frequent.

Advice on the issue of hearing aids and supervision of their use is a duty which could be undertaken by an audiologist. It is recommended that an audiologist should work in conjunction with one or more peripatetic teachers of the deaf.

It has been suggested that the work of a peripatetic teacher should be concerned to a considerable extent with children of nursery and infant school age and parent guidance. This part of their work would be mainly preventive, and aimed at avoiding educational retardation and social maladjustment in later years. By close liaison with ordinary schools, units for nursery/infant and junior school children, where these are provided, and special schools, they could assist in making decisions as to placement. In the case of children considered suitable for ordinary schooling their duties would consist of follow-up procedures, school visit-ing, and parent and teacher guidance. It is not felt that a system of peripatetic teaching can, at the present time, take the place of special schooling for a great number of those children for whom it is now considered necessary. Such children are often widely scattered in any given area, of considerable age range, and of very varied nature with regard to their individual difficulties. Unless a great many peripatetic teachers were provided, the amount of help each child could receive would be most inadequate.

The extent to which peripatetic teachers would be able to assist with remedial teaching of retarded children would again depend on the number of children they have under their care. It is obvious that serious educational retardation, such as has been observed in some cases in this study, requires more intensive teaching than can be given by a teacher only available for a short period each week.

Educational retardation due to impaired hearing can only be overcome by a long-term scheme of early ascertainment, followed by detailed diagnosis and careful decisions as to placement.

The appointment of an audiologist and peripatetic teachers of the deaf is suggested as a preliminary to the opening of units attached to ordinary schools for young deaf children, when these are projected. In this way detailed knowledge of the number of children likely to benefit from such provision could be obtained, and a decision made as to the most suitable areas, and schools, in which to open units. It has been pointed out that units for nursery and infant school children could serve a useful purpose as diagnostic and educational centres for children whose subsequent education might be either in ordinary schools or special schools. These units would be of great assistance in the making of decisions as to eventual school placement. There is also a strong argument in their favour in that they would avoid the sending of very young children away from their homes to residential special schools. In some cases, distance of travel might prevent a young child being enrolled in a unit, though experience in existing units has shown that travelling distance is not a major obstacle. However, a peripatetic teacher would be in a position to give greater attention to young children unable to attend a unit, who would be his especial responsibility.

Units attached to ordinary schools for children of junior school age are recommended in areas where a sufficient number of children, for whom such provision is considered suitable, can be brought together. It is suggested that unit placement for children of this age should be thought of as a short-term arrangement, i.e. for children who could eventually return to the ordinary schools. These would be children who, by reason of their hearing impairment, educational attainments and linguistic and social development need a period of more specialised help than can be given in an ordinary school.

This study has attempted to describe some of the difficulties which face children with impaired hearing and to outline means of combating them. It has shown that impaired hearing is a very serious handicap, which can have widespread effects on the educational and social progress of children in the ordinary schools. As to those children who can best benefit from ordinary schooling, this is always a matter for an individual decision in the case of each child. Such a decision cannot be hurriedly made or made on the basis of a single factor.

With regard to future policy, it is clear from this study that not enough is yet being done for children already in ordinary schools, for any immediate change of policy in the present system of special education for children with impaired hearing. It is true that a question mark hangs over the system of segregation for very deaf children. In principle, one must accept that segregation is not an ideal policy, in view of the fact that handicapped children must eventually take their place in society. But to suggest sweeping changes in the special school system at this stage would be ill-advised. In the years ahead it may well be that more detailed attention can be given to solving the problem of how to give children with severe hearing impairment adequate education and, at the same time, fuller opportunities to mix socially with unhandicapped children. Experiments are in progress in the U.S.A. in part-time ordinary schooling for such children, in a system of close liaison between ordinary schools, audiology clinics and special schools.[1] Similar experiments in this country would be welcomed, but it would be a pity if they were to supersede the setting up, in the country as a whole, of more thorough arrangements for the ascertainment, diagnosis and treatment of impaired hearing.

[1] McLaughlin, H. F., 'Integration of Deaf Children into Hearing Society', *The Modern Educational Treatment of Deafness*, Paper 11.

# BIBLIOGRAPHY

Advisory Council on Education in Scotland, Report of *Pupils who are Defective in Hearing* (H.M.S.O., 1950).

BALLANTYNE, J. C., *Deafness* (Churchill, 1960).

Board of Education, Report of Committee of Inquiry into Problems Relating to Children with Defective Hearing (H.M.S.O., 1938).

BOWLEY, A. H., *The Young Handicapped Child* (Livingstone, 1957).

BRERETON, B. LE GAY, *The Schooling of Children with Impaired Hearing* (Commonwealth Office of Education, Sydney, 1957).

CAPLAN, G., *Emotional Problems of Early Childhood* (Basic Books Inc., New York, 1955).

CRUICKSHANK, W. M., *The Psychology of Exceptional Children and Youth* (Prentice-Hall, 1955).

CURRY, E. T., 'Are Teachers Good Judges of Pupils' Hearing?', *Journal of Exceptional Children*, Vol. 21, 1954.

DALE, D. M. C., 'The Possibility of Providing Extensive Auditory Experience for Severely and Profoundly Deaf Children by the Use of Hearing Aids', unpublished Thesis, Christie Library, University of Manchester, 1958.

DAVIS, H. (ed.), *Hearing and Deafness* (Murray Hill Books, New York, 1957).

DICARLO, L. M., 'The Deaf and Hard of Hearing', *Review of Educational Research*, Vol. 29, No. 5, December 1959.

DUNSDON, M. I., *The Education of Cerebral Palsied Children* (Newnes Educational Publishing, 1951).

EWING, I. and A. W. G., *Speech and the Deaf Child* (Manchester University Press, 1954).

EWING, A. W. G. (ed.), *Educational Guidance and the Deaf Child* (Manchester University Press, 1957).

—— *New Opportunities for Deaf Children* (University of London Press, 1958).

—— (ed.), *The Modern Educational Treatment of Deafness* (Manchester University Press, 1959).

GARDNER, W., Report of Committee on Hard of Hearing Children, *Hearing News*, 1950.

HARDY, W. G., 'The Assessment of Hearing in Children and an Interpretation of the Findings', *The Modern Educational Treatment of Deafness*, Paper 18.

HARRISON, K., 'The Aetiology of Deafness in Childhood', *Modern Educational Treatment of Deafness*, Paper 7.

HIRSH, I. J., *The Measurement of Hearing* (McGraw-Hill, New York, 1952).

HOCH, P. H., and ZUBIN, J., *Psychopathology of Childhood* (Grune and Stratton, 1955).

HODGSON, K. W., *The Deaf and their Problems* (Watts and Co., 1953).

ILLINGWORTH, R. S. (ed.), *Recent Advances in Cerebral Palsy* (Churchill, 1958).

JOHN, J. E. J., 'Audiology Clinics', *Medical Officer*, Vol. 105, No. 3, 1961.

JOHNSEN, S., 'Incidence and Correlation between Aetiology and Audiometric Pattern', *Journal of Laryngology and Otology*, 1957.

KARELITZ, S., *When Your Child is Ill* (Jonathan Cape, 1958).

LING, D., 'Provision of Services for Deaf Children in Reading', *Teacher of the Deaf*, Vol. 58, 343.

—— 'The Education and General Background of Children with Defective Hearing in Reading', Cambridge Institute of Education Library, 1959.

MCLAUGHLIN, H. F., 'The Integration of Deaf Children into Hearing Society', *The Modern Educational Treatment of Deafness*, Paper 11.

Ministry of Education, *Special Educational Treatment* (H.M.S.O., 1946).

—— *Education of the Handicapped Pupil* (H.M.S.O., 1956).

—— *The Health of the School Child* (1954–5, 1956–7 and 1958–9) (H.M.S.O.).

—— *Education in England and Wales* (Report and Statistics, 1959) (H.M.S.O., 1960).

MINSKI, L., *Deafness, Mutism and Mental Deficiency in Children* (Heinemann, 1957).

National College of Teachers of the Deaf, 'List of Schools, Units, etc., for the Deaf and Partially Deaf', 1960.

NEWBY, H. A., *Audiology* (Vision Press, 1959).

ROBINSON, J. B., *Report on the Care of the Deaf* (National Deaf Children's Society, 1958).

SCOTT-BROWN, W. G., *Methods of Examination in E.N.T.* (Butterworth, 1954).

Scottish Council for Research in Education, *Hearing Defects of School Children* (University of London Press, 1956).

SHERIDAN, M. D., *The Child's Hearing for Speech* (Methuen, 1948).

SIEGENTHALER, B., 'The Use of Hearing Aids by Public School Children', *Archives of Otolaryngology*, 1958.

Society of Teachers of the Deaf, 'Memorandum on Units for Deaf and Partially Deaf Children', *Teacher of the Deaf*, Vol. 58, No. 345.

STEVENSON, A. C., and CHEESEMAN, E. A., 'Hereditary Deaf Mutism with particular reference to Northern Ireland', *Annals of Human Genetics*, Vol. 20, Part III, 1956.

STOTT, D. H., *The Social Adjustment of Children* (University of London Press, 1958).

STRENG, A. (ed.), *Hearing Therapy for Children* (Grune and Stratton, 1958).

TRAVIS, L. (ed.), *Handbook of Speech Pathology* (Appleton-Century-Crofts, 1957).

# INDEX

acoustic feed-back, 62
acoustics, 14, 55, 61, 62, 83, 112, 113
Advisory Council on Education in
    Scotland, 12, 16, 23
aetiology of deafness, 10, 12, 14, 20, 39,
    40, 41, 97
age of onset, 28, 30, 31, 40, 47, 49, 50,
    106, 109, 112
age of first referral, 28, 29
arithmetic, 1, 8, 14, 15, 44, 45, 102, 103
articulation of speech, 47–52, 101, 110
ascertainment, 3, 6, 22, 25, 28, 29, 30,
    78, 79, 97, 109–12, 115
attitudes
    of parents, 60, 62, 66, 69, 71, 75, 77,
        84
    of teachers, 63, 67, 80, 82, 83, 86, 87,
        105, 113
audiogram
    availability of, 32
    interpretation of, 33
    pattern of, 32–9, 57
    pure tone, 47
    speech, 47
audiologist, 92, 93, 110, 114, 115
audiology
    clinics, 4, 6, 7, 25, 66, 76, 79, 110, 111
    diploma in, 93
audiometry
    of age groups, 5, 110
    conflicting results in, 30, 32, 33
    gramophone, 109
    pure tone, 5, 47, 110
    of risk groups, 41
    screening tests, 24
    speech, 47, 52, 53, 55, 100, 110
average hearing impairment
    defined, 5
    disadvantages of, 32

Brereton, B. Le Gay, 14, 51

case histories, 29, 30, 33–9, 67–76
causation of deafness, see aetiology
cerebral palsy, 20
Cheshire, County of, 2, 3, 4, 6, 7, 24,
    25, 26, 58, 95–108, 111, 112

classification, 9, 10, 96
comprehension of spoken language,
    14, 47, 52–7, 99
conductive deafness, 10–12, 22–6, 37–9,
    49
    defined, 11
    incidence of, 22–6

deafness, see hearing impairment
degree of hearing impairment, 31–3,
    49, 54, 56, 82, 97, 98, 112
Department of Audiology and Educa-
    tion of the Deaf, University of
    Manchester, 4, 6, 7, 8, 93
diagnosis
    delayed, 28, 29, 74
    differential, 111

educational attainment, 1, 8, 12, 15, 43,
    44, 102–4
    arithmetic, 44, 102
    reading, 43, 102
educational placement, 28, 29, 107, 108
educational provision, 85–94, 109–16

familial deafness, 39, 40
Fife Survey, 1, 13, 15, 17, 23

Glasgow, City of, 24

Hampshire, County of, 60
health visitors, 109
hearing aid centres, 59, 60
hearing aids, 12, 21–3, 42, 43, 47, 58–
    63, 66, 67, 83, 84, 92, 100, 112, 113
    commercial, 58, 59
    ear moulds, 62
    inductance loops, 113, 114
    issue of, 59, 113
    knowledge by teachers of, 63
    training in use of, 113
    transistor, 22, 43
hearing impairment
    age of onset of, 28, 30, 31, 40, 47,
        49, 50, 106, 109, 112
    ascertainment of, 3, 6, 22, 25, 28, 29,
        30, 78, 79, 97, 109–12, 115

hearing impairment (*cont.*)
  average, 5, 31, 32
  bilateral, 18, 22
  causes of, *see* aetiology
  classification of, 9, 10, 96
  conductive, 10–12, 22–6, 37–9, 49
  degree of, 31–3, 49, 54, 56, 82, 97, 98, 112
  detection by teachers of, 110
  familial, 39, 40
  grades of, 9, 10, 96
  hereditary, 39, 40
  incidence of, 16–26
  indications of, 78, 79, 110
  lipreading and, 31, 40, 47, 52, 53, 56, 69, 82
  pattern of, 33–8, 57
  perceptive, 10, 11, 18, 21, 25, 40, 49, 50, 69
  significant, 5, 13
  type of, 33–9
  unilateral, 13, 21, 24
high frequency consonants, 50, 110

incidence of hearing impairment, 16–26
inductance loop, 113, 114
integration, 1, 14, 51, 89, 90, 116
intelligence
  assessment of, 45
  distribution of, 46, 104
  performance tests of, 46
  verbal tests of, 46

Johnsen, Steen, 18, 21

late diagnosis, 28, 29, 74
Ling, D., 15
lipreading, 31, 40, 47, 52, 53, 56, 69, 82
  classes, 13
  dependence on, 56, 81
London County Council, 18
loop, inductance, 113, 114

Medresco hearing aid, 22, 58, 113
meningitis, 30, 41
MJ Word Lists, 8, 55, 100

National Health Service, 22, 59

occupation centres, 19, 21
ordinary schools
  incidence of hearing impairment in, 21–6
  units attached to, 3, 18, 85–91, 115

otitis media, 10

parent guidance, 60, 76, 84, 92, 93, 114
pattern of hearing impairment, 33–8, 57
perceptive deafness, 10, 18, 21–5, 40
  defined, 11
  high frequency, 32, 33–8, 49, 50, 53, 69
peripatetic teachers, 2, 60, 77, 79, 83, 91–4, 113, 114
pre-school children, 25, 57, 92, 109, 111
previous inquiries, 9–15
private schools, 25, 26
psychologist, 111

Raven's Matrices Test, 8, 45, 46, 104
Reading, County Borough of, 15, 22, 85
record forms, 89, 111
Report of 1938 Committee of Inquiry, 3, 5, 9–11, 16, 21, 23
rubella, 14

Scottish Council for Research in Education, 1, 13, 16
screening tests of hearing, 13, 24, 25, 109
Sheridan, M. D., 11, 12
sign language, 102
significant hearing impairment, defined, 5
social adjustment, 8, 64–77, 105
social worker, 76
special schools, 16–20, 95–108
  age of entry to, 88
speech
  articulation of, 47–52, 101
  defects in, 50, 110
speech audiometry, 47, 52, 53, 55, 100
Stott, D. H., 65
sweep frequency test, 13, 24, 109

training colleges, 63, 84
type of hearing impairment, 33–9

undiagnosed hearing impairment, 6, 12, 13, 111
  reasons for, 29
units for partially deaf children, 3, 18, 85–91, 115

Warrington, County Borough of, 4
Wechsler Intelligence Scale, 88
whisper tests, 29

# Date Due

| | | | |
|---|---|---|---|
| 6-15-68 | | | |
| APR 07 77 | | | |
| APR 14 77 | | | |
| DEC 0 9 2004 | | | |
| | | | |
| | | | |
| | | | |
| | | | |
| | | | |
| | | | |
| | | | |
| | | | |
| | | | |
| | | | |
| | | | |
| | | | |